the cutting book

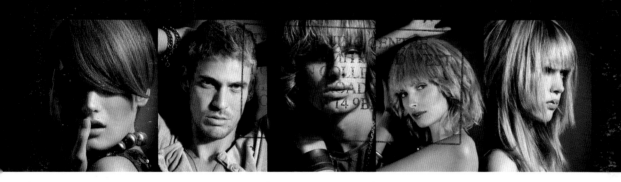

Habia SERIES

HAIRDRESSING

Mahogany Hairdressing: Steps to Cutting, Colouring and Finishing Hair *Martin Gannon and Richard Thompson*
Mahogany Hairdressing: Advanced Looks *Richard Thompson and Martin Gannon*
Professional Men's Hairdressing *Guy Kremer and Jacki Wadeson*
The Art of Dressing Long Hair *Guy Kremer and Jacki Wadeson*
Patrick Cameron: Dressing Long Hair *Patrick Cameron and Jacki Wadeson*
Patrick Cameron: Dressing Long Hair Book 2 *Patrick Cameron*
Bridal Hair *Pat Dixon and Jacki Wadeson*
Trevor Sorbie: Visions in Hair *Kris Sorbie and Jacki Wadeson*
The Total Look: The Style Guide for Hair and Make-Up Professionals *Ian Mistlin*
Art of Hair Colouring *David Adams and Jacki Wadeson*
Begin Hairdressing: The Official Guide to Level 1 2e *Martin Green*
Hairdressing – The Foundations: The Official Guide to Level 2 5e *Leo Palladino* (contribution Jane Farr)
Professional Hairdressing: The Official Guide to Level 3 4e *Martin Green, Lesley Kimber and Leo Palladino*
Men's Hairdressing: Traditional and Modern Barbering 2e *Maurice Lister*
African-Caribbean Hairdressing 2e *Sandra Gittens*
Salon Management *Martin Green*
eXtensions: The Official Guide to Hair Extensions *Theresa Bullock*
Trevor Sorbie: The Bridal Hair Book *Trevor Sorbie and Jacki Wadeson*
The Colour Book: The Official Guide to Colour for Levels 2 and 3 *Tracey Lloyd with Christine McMillan-Bodell*
The World of Hair Colour *Dr John Gray*
Hairdressing – The Foundations: Lecturer's Resource Pack, The Official Guide to Level 2 *Jane Farr*

BEAUTY THERAPY

Beauty Basics – The Official Guide to Level 1 *Lorraine Nordmann*
Beauty Therapy – The Foundations: The Official Guide to Level 2 4e *Lorraine Nordmann*
Professional Beauty Therapy: The Official Guide to Level 3 2e *Lorraine Nordmann, Lorraine Williamson, Pamela Linforth and Jo Crowder*
Aromatherapy for the Beauty Therapist *Valerie Ann Worwood*
Indian Head Massage 2e *Muriel Burnham-Airey and Adele O'Keefe*
The Official Guide to Body Massage 2e *Adele O'Keefe*
An Holistic Guide to Anatomy and Physiology *Tina Parsons*
The Encyclopedia of Nails 2e *Jacqui Jefford and Anne Swain*
Nail Artistry *Jacqui Jefford, Sue Marsh and Anne Swain*
The Complete Nail Technician 2e *Marian Newman*
The World of Skin Care: A Scientific Companion *Dr John Gray*
Safety in the Salon *Elaine Almond*
An Holistic Guide to Reflexology *Tina Parsons*
Nutrition: A Practical Approach *Suzanne Le Quesne*
An Holistic Guide to Massage *Tina Parsons*
The Spa Book: The Official Guide to Spa Therapy *Jane Crebbin-Bailey, Dr John Harcup and John Harrington*
The Art of Nails: A Comprehensive Style Guide to Nail Treatments and Nail Art *Jacqui Jefford*
The Complete Guide to Make-up *Suzanne LeQuesne*
The Essential Guide to Holistic and Complementary Therapy *Helen Beckmann and Suzanne LeQuesne*
Hands On Sports Therapy *Kevin Ward*
Manicure, Pedicure and Advanced Nail Techniques *Elaine Almond*
Complete Make-up Artist: Working in Film, Fashion, Television and Theatre 2e *Penny Delamar*

the cutting book

THE OFFICIAL GUIDE TO CUTTING FOR S/NVQ LEVELS 2 AND 3

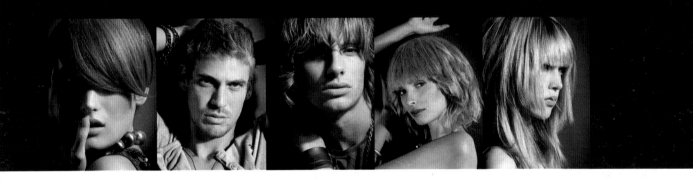

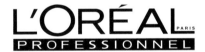

JANE GOLDSBRO AND ELAINE WHITE

City&Guilds

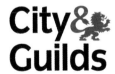

Australia • Canada • Mexico • Singapore • Spain • United Kingdom • United States

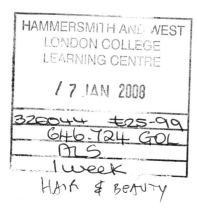

THOMSON
™

The Cutting Book

Jane Goldsbro and Elaine White

Publishing Director	**Commissioning Editor**	**Development Editor**
John Yates	Melody Dawes	Elizabeth Catford
Production Editor	**Manufacturing Manager**	**Marketing Manager**
Alissa Chappell	Helen Mason	Leo Stanley
Typesetter	**Production Controller**	**Printer**
Graphicraft	Maeve Healy	Canale, Italy
Cover Design	**Text Design**	
MCT Creative Ltd., Hampshire	Design Deluxe, Bath, UK	

British Library Cataloguing-in-Publication Data
A catalogue record for this book is available from the British Library

This publication has been developed by Thomson Learning. It is intended as a method of studying for the Habia qualifications. Thomson Learning has taken all reasonable care in the preparation of this publication but Thomson Learning and the City and Guilds of London Institute accept no liability howsoever in respect of any breach of the rights of any third party howsoever occasioned or damage caused to any third party as a result of the use of this publication.

contents

dedication

Jane Goldsbro

I would like to dedicate this book to my husband Alan and to my parents for their continual love and support whilst I was writing.

Elaine White

I would like to dedicate this book to my husband Graham and to my children Jenna and James for their constant love and support.

what can the cutting book do for you?

If you ask any new entrant to the hairdressing industry, they will tell you that the skill they most want to learn is how to cut hair. Yet haircutting is not just about reducing the length of hair – it's much, much more. *The Cutting Book* will help you with all the background knowledge that you need to know in order to create the most amazing looks for your clients.

Haircutting can be creative yet structured, and innovative yet methodical. With this in mind *The Cutting Book* takes you through all the haircuts, both in words and pictures, that you will use within your S/NVQ at Levels 2 and 3. And, beyond this, it takes you into looks that can be created which are only limited by the boundaries of your own imagination.

The Cutting Book includes useful tips, step-by-step images and expert advice about how to cut hair, as well as interesting activities designed especially to match the stage you have reached in your training that will help you retain the knowledge you need for your qualification. There is an accompanying CD-ROM that provides another dimension for learning about haircutting.

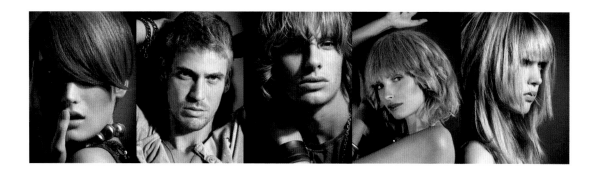

acknowledgements

Jane Goldsbro and Elaine White would like to thank Lizzie Catford and Melody Dawes for their support and guidance during the writing of the book, Gaynor Hodge and Shonali Bandopadhyay for the support from L'Oréal and Jackie Holian and the team from Habia for all their help.

The publisher would also like to thank:

Alan and Karen Simpson,
   Contemporary Salons North East
Alan Edwards
American Dream
Andis
Andrew Barton
Andrew Collinge
Anita Cox
Anne McGuigan Art Team, Leighton
   Buzzard
Anne Veck, Anne Veck Hair
Anthony Mascolo
Antoinette Beenders, Aveda
Asahi scissors
BaByliss
BLM Health
Bruno Miarli, Altered Image
Cheynes Hairdressing
Chubb Fire Ltd
David Johnson, Brave New World
Denman
Dr Andrew Wright
Dr H.M. Beck
Dr John Gray
Dr P. Marazzi/Science Photo Library
Ellisons

Excellent Edges Ltd
Frank Bisson
Gary Gill
Getty Images
Habia
Helen Ward, Richard Ward Hair
   and Metrospa
John Burbage/Science photo
   library
Kasho scissors
Keith Hall, Creative Team
Mark Hill
Mediscan
Mucktaro Kargbo, MK Hair Studio
Nikki Froud Artistic Team
Peter Prosser Hairdressing
Picture-desk image library
Rand Rocket
Redken
Richard Ward
SAFE-System
Saks
Susan Hall, Reds Hair and Beauty
Toni & Guy
Vicky Turner, Goldsworthy's
Wahl (UK) ltd

Habia foreword

I am delighted that two people whom I have known and worked with for a long time have joined forces to write this book.

Elaine White and Jane Goldsbro are authorities in their field and their input into the hairdressing industry is immense. Through their work with Habia they push forward the standards for hairdressing education worldwide.

Elaine has over 30 years experience within the industry, including over 16 years as a hairdressing lecturer and course team leader. Her current role as Senior Development Manager for Habia has been pivotal to many developments by Habia, including the new young apprenticeship. Elaine is a true professional whose exacting standards and dedication to her work has enabled her to focus on the end product with outstanding results.

Jane has over 25 years experience within the hairdressing industry, including salon management, educator and now Director of Standards and Qualifications at Habia. The commitment she has to her work is phenomenal. From writing standards, managing people and relationships with partners to international development, her wide vision means that she has an impressive ability to see the steps needed to achieve an end result.

Both women have a huge passion for their craft and this book is testament to that.

I cannot think of two more qualified people to be at the heart of this book.

Alan Goldsbro
Habia
Chief Executive Officer

about the authors

Elaine White With a driving passion, Elaine White has expanded on her 30 years experience in the hairdressing industry by implementing some of the most influential programmes within work-based learning.

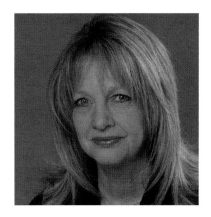

Throughout her career, Elaine has been directly involved in researching processes and developing systems that have raised standards within the hair and beauty industry. Elaine has contributed massively to the development of structures in UK and international hair and beauty education, which are renowned throughout the world. Throughout her career her passion for learning and development, not only for herself but for others, took her into the challenging world of further and higher education. Here she spent more than 16 years as an educator in both Lincolnshire and Nottinghamshire, before joining Habia in 2001 as Senior Development Manager.

Her role as Senior Development Manager allows her to work with a diverse range of stakeholders, encompassing employers, schools, colleges of further education, private training providers and universities. This has allowed Elaine to lead the development of innovative programmes including the Young Apprenticeships, Apprenticeships and Foundation Degrees, setting the standard for hair and beauty education from school pupils to university graduates. One of the most rewarding projects was to research the incidence of dyslexia in the hairdressing industry that culminated a presentation to an invited group at the House of Lords, the home of the upper chamber in the UK Parliament.

This invaluable experience has enabled Elaine to develop and update education over all six sectors of Habia's portfolio in hair, beauty, nails, spa, barbering and African-type hair. Her knowledge and experience has been further recognised through the appointment of the standard-setting body representative for the Apprenticeship Approval Group for England and Wales.

If this wasn't enough, Elaine is also an associate inspector for the Adult Learning Inspectorate. Her passion for quality is paramount and clearly evident through her work.

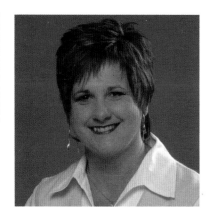

Jane Goldsbro A qualified hairdresser since 1982, Jane is one of the most influential educators in hair and beauty today. Her skills in developing the structure of UK hair and beauty education are renowned throughout the world.

Jane's early career as a hairdresser took her through a formative path where she ran salons and worked for some of the best companies and key influencers in the field of education, such as Alan International. At Redken she worked as one of their top technicians.

At an early stage of her career, Jane was a regional winner of the L'Oréal Colour Trophy at the tender age of 17; this led her to start a teaching career at her local college. However, the deep-rooted commitment to continue learning saw Jane taking on her biggest challenge when she began work at Habia.

In 1992 Jane started work at Habia as Development Manager for Hairdressing and within four years had risen to Director of Standards and Qualifications. This role saw her take on bigger challenges every year. Not only did Jane enhance the development of hairdressing education, she began to expand Habia's remit into beauty therapy. Since those heady days of endless development meetings, running standards workshops and training international educators in Habia techniques, Jane still found time to develop her skills.

An established writer of technical material for Habia, Jane is also the author of two hairdressing study guides for Thomson Learning, the leading publisher in hair and beauty. Her expertise in training and assessing has been picked up by well-known awarding bodies such as City & Guilds and at the inception of a new regulatory regime by the UK government in training, Jane became one of the first inspectors for the Adult Learning Inspectorate.

Her role at Habia as Director of Standards and Qualifications now covers all six sectors of Habia's portfolio in hair, beauty, nails, spa, barbering and African-type hair. She is responsible for setting the standard for hair and beauty education from school leavers to university graduates.

Truly, one of the most knowledgeable hair and beauty educators in the world.

about the stylists

Andy Smith Formerly Artistic Director for the John Carne Group, Andy Smith is now the Guildford Salon Manager. Although only 25 years old, Andy has already achieved a great deal in his career, including winning the prestigious L'Oréal Colour Trophy 2004 and winning the Men's Image Award 2005, both with colleague Harriet White. Andy has also done session styling and editorial work for publications including *Vogue, Marie Claire, Glamour* and *Cosmopolitan* as well as television work for Channel Four and GMTV.

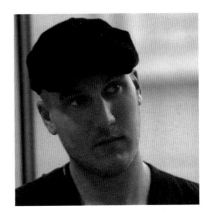

This broad experience has opened many doors for Andy, enabling him to work on high-profile events such as London Fashion Week and the famous St Martin's College of Fashion Student Shows. Andy has also represented the John Carne brand at many international and UK shows around the world. Education is another area that Andy is heavily involved in and has a great passion for. He has worked on numerous large-scale training events and seminars for L'Oréal, KMS and Redken as well as taking a leading role in all in-salon training for the John Carne Group.

Carly Aplin began her career in hairdressing as a 15-year-old Saturday girl, continuing her training and working in the north-west, before joining Cutting Room Creative in June 2006. She has quickly been promoted on to the C.R.C. Art Team and is Assistant trainer at the salon.

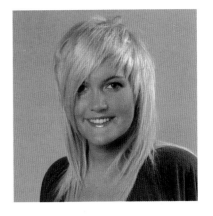

Carly has already had a varied and exciting career, winning Talent Spotting in 2004 and joining L'Oréal's ID Team in 2005. This opened many doors for her and to date she has worked on a number of shows for Central St Martin's Graduate Fashion Week, the BAFTAs and Salon International, for both the Fellowship and *Hairdressers Journal*.

She has just won a coveted place on the Fellowships Project X and looks set to continue her meteoric rise.

Claire Morley, 22, of Contemporary Guisborough is one of the salon chain's rising stars. She is already an award-winning session stylist, winning the Tigi Inspirational Youth Award earlier this year in addition to being named a national finalist in the L'Oréal Colour Trophy Next Generation Award.

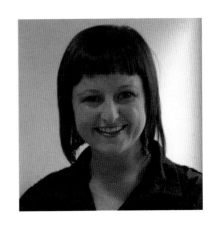

She joined the Contemporary group four years ago and divides her time between working in the Guisborough salon, shooting with the Contemporary Art Team and at shows, as well as working with the Tigi Youth Artistic Team.

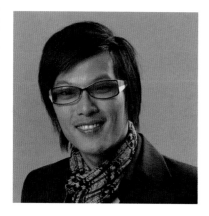

Herman Ho is part of the Headmasters Artistic Team. The maintains a strong column in the salon whilst being a member of the art team. This means Herman works on and off stage regularly, creates trend predictions with the Art Team and also educates stylists throughout the group.

Herman's off stage work has included The British Style Awards, London Fashion Week 2003/4/5, Graduate Fashion Week 2004/5, and the London Fashion Forum. He has also worked on TV shows for MTV, VH1 and Sky One. In 2003 Herman won the prestigious L'Oréal Colour Trophy for his men's image. The winning image was a rebellious grown-out mohican with contrasting blonde highlights on black. Herman was also a regional finalist for L'Oréal Talent Spotting 2003.

Herman joined Headmasters in January 2002 from his native Hong Kong where he trained as a hairdresser from the age of 17 in the family business. Now with over 10 years experience and prestigious industry awards under his belt, Herman is excited about his future, 'The hair industry is going through such an exhilarating time at the moment and it holds so many fantastic opportunities for someone like me, I am really looking forward to the years to come.'

For press information and artistic images from Herman Ho please contact Laura Hinton at Headmasters on 0208 296 6472 or e-mail laura@hmhair.co.uk

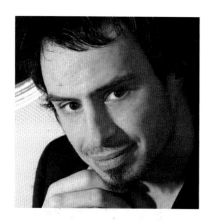

Jonny Engstrom is the Art Director of celebrity stylist Guy Kremer and travels the world working on seminars, hair exhibitions and photo shoots. He has worked for the Guy Kremer Hair Salon, based in Winchester, for nine years.

He is a very likeable, laid back character with a quirky sense of humour and an infectious laugh, which erupts every so often.

A firm favourite with top designers, fashion and beauty editors, Engstrom is regularly requested to work for the national newspapers such as the *Daily* and *Sunday Express*, *Evening Standard*, *Happy Magazine* fashion pages, top magazines such as *FHM*, *Shine* and *Eve* and wedding magazines *Bride*, *You and Your Wedding* and *Bride and Groom*. In February 2006 he went to Thailand for a shoot with the *Daily Express*.

He has been twice requested for Selfridges window designs and appears in the film *Blow Dry*.

Winner of the 1999 L'Oreal Men's Image Award, nominated for Southern Hairdresser of the year 1998 and Winner of the 2001 L'Oréal Colour Trophy Grand Final for the Guy Kremer Salon.

Jonny regularly works for L'Oréal Professionnel teaching advanced hairdressing to students, in particular bridal hair, and during 2005/2006 he has travelled to India, Australia, Turkey and Greece.

Lyndsey Brockway has worked for The Level Hair Salon Group for eight years. She gained a wealth of experience from session styling at 'Pure Fashion Week' (four times) and from being part of the Team of London Graduates Fashion Week (twice). Lyndsey says 'I love the buzz you get from the pressure of catwalk styling, which enables me to carry more enthusiasm and passion back into the salon on a daily basis.'

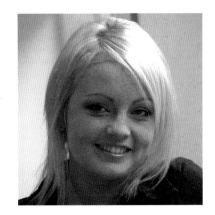

Having now been made Group Artistic Director, Lyndsey's responsibilities range from updating images in the Salons, organising photo shoots, and in-house competitions, to external activities with L'Oréal and the major fashion houses.

This year her goal is to raise the profile of Level both in the trade and commercially through photographic collections and more session work.

Phill Gallagher is the Artistic Director for Headmasters luxury high street salons. Phill's role includes session and editorial work as well as working with the Senior Artistic Team to create trend predictions, education and training throughout the salon group, as well as running a busy salon column.

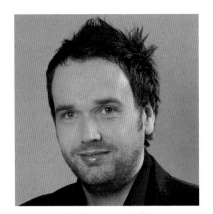

Phill is in constant demand for shows on and off stage and has recently worked on London Fashion Week, the Irish L'Oréal Colour Trophy Show and was the Co-Director of hair at Graduate Fashion Week 2005.

Phill's work includes editorials from *The Sunday Times Style* to *Elle*. Phill has worked backstage on fashion legends such as Kate Moss, Linda Evangelista, Erin O'Connor, Lizzie Jagger and Lily Cole, and pop icons Dannii Minogue, Kelly Osbourne and Jamelia.

Tiziana Dimarcelli originally from Italy, but trained in Switzerland and has been working at the Trevor Sorbie salon for several years where she has learned and contributed to new techniques. Tiziana is joint head of education at Trevor Sorbie and enjoys working on shows, seminars, teaching and photoshoots. Tiziana says 'It was interesting to work on something new, which was a challenge and a very good experience.'

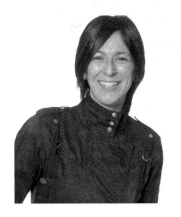

The authors and Publisher would like to thank Saks and Andrew Barton for the use of the chapter opener images which are all from the current Saks cut and colour collection for 2007.

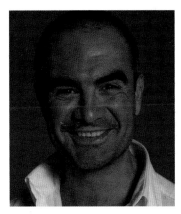

The collection stems from months of research by the Saks Art Team, headed by current British Hairdresser of the Year and resident hair celebrity on 10 Years Younger, Andrew Barton.

Andrew says: High Definition is inspired by international catwalk trends and the woman's needs and desires, rejecting over-formal, structured hair for a mix of uptown glitz and downtown chic. It's a noticeable shift in style, texture, shape, cut and colour. Looks in the collection range from fringed crop to swishing bob, from lazy layers to retro rock gothess.

about the book

The Cutting Book relates to the structures for S/NVQ Levels 2 and 3 and to the current Habia National Occupational Standards for hairdressing and barbering.

The Cutting Book is related to the following units:

H6   Cut hair using basic techniques

H7   Cut hair using basic barbering techniques

H27 Create a variety of looks using a combination of cutting techniques

H21 Create a variety of looks using barbering techniques

When cutting hair you also need to have knowledge to work hygienically and safely, how to communicate effectively and how to provide the correct advice to your clients. So *The Cutting Book* also relates to the following units:

G1   Ensure your own actions reduce risks to health and safety

G7   Advise and consult with clients

G9   Provide hairdressing consultation services

One whole chapter of the book is dedicated to providing clear step-by-step coverage for a range of cutting looks required for S/NVQ Level 2 and Level 3.

Features within the chapters

Each chapter of the book is full of lively examples and full colour illustrations plus the following carefully constructed features to aid your learning process:

Quotes Each of the seven chapters begins with a quote from an exceptionally talented hairdresser. The quotes will provide you with an indication of what you can find within the chapter.

Learning objectives The learning objectives are stated in each of the chapters. They outline what you can expect to have learned by the end of the chapter.

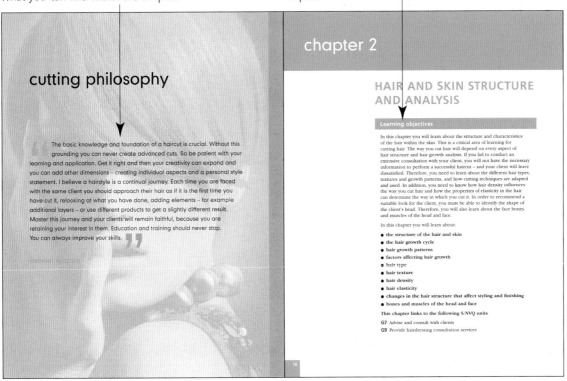

cutting philosophy

The basic knowledge and foundation of a haircut is crucial. Without this grounding you can never create advanced cuts. So be patient with your learning and application. Get it right and then your creativity can expand and you can add other dimensions – creating individual aspects and a personal style statement. I believe a hairstyle is a continual journey. Each time you are faced with the same client you should approach their hair as if it is the first time you have cut it, relooking at what you have done, adding elements – for example additional layers – or use different products to get a slightly different result. Master this journey and your clients will remain faithful, because you are retaining your interest in them. Education and training should never stop. You can always improve your skills.

ANTHONY MASCOLO

chapter 2

HAIR AND SKIN STRUCTURE AND ANALYSIS

Learning objectives

In this chapter you will learn about the structure and characteristics of the hair within the skin. This is a critical area of learning for cutting hair. The way you cut hair will depend on every aspect of hair structure and hair growth analysis. If you fail to conduct an extensive consultation with your client, you will not have the necessary information to perform a successful haircut – and your client will leave dissatisfied. Therefore, you need to learn about the different hair types, textures and growth patterns, and how cutting techniques are adapted and used. In addition, you need to know how hair density influences the way you cut hair and how the properties of elasticity in the hair can determine the way in which you cut it. In order to recommend a suitable look for the client, you must be able to identify the shape of the client's head. Therefore, you will also learn about the face bones and muscles of the head and face.

In this chapter you will learn about:

- the structure of the hair and skin
- the hair growth cycle
- hair growth patterns
- factors affecting hair growth
- hair type
- hair texture
- hair density
- hair elasticity
- changes in the hair structure that affect styling and finishing
- bones and muscles of the head and face

This chapter links to the following S/NVQ units

G7 Advise and consult with clients
G9 Provide hairdressing consultation services

18

Introduction The introduction outlines the areas of learning and sets the context for the chapter.

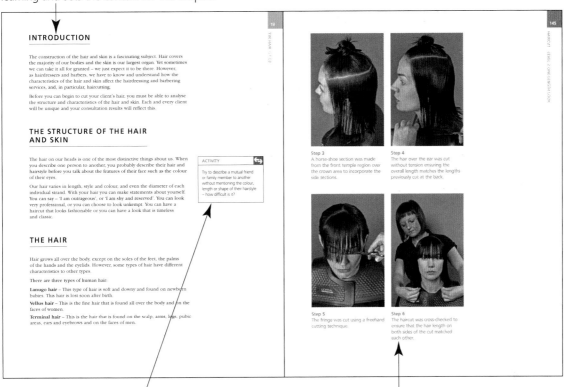

INTRODUCTION

19 · THE HAIR & SKIN

The construction of the hair and skin is a fascinating subject. Hair covers the majority of our bodies and the skin is our largest organ. Yet sometimes we can take it all for granted – we just expect it to be there. However, as hairdressers and barbers, we have to know and understand how the characteristics of the hair and skin affect the hairdressing and barbering services, and, in particular, haircutting.

Before you can begin to cut your client's hair, you must be able to analyse the structure and characteristics of the hair and skin. Each and every client will be unique and your consultation results will reflect this.

THE STRUCTURE OF THE HAIR AND SKIN

The hair on our heads is one of the most distinctive things about us. When you describe one person to another, you probably describe their hair and hairstyle before you talk about the features of their face such as the colour of their eyes.

Our hair varies in length, style and colour, and even the diameter of each individual strand. With your hairstyle you can make statements about yourself. You can say – 'I am outrageous', or 'I am shy and reserved'. You can look very professional, or you can choose to look unkempt. You can have a haircut that looks fashionable or you can have a look that is timeless and classic.

THE HAIR

Hair grows all over the body, except on the soles of the feet, the palms of the hands and the eyelids. However, some types of hair have different characteristics to other types.

There are three types of human hair:

Lanugo hair – This type of hair is soft and downy and found on newborn babies. This hair is lost soon after birth.
Vellus hair – This is the fine hair that is found all over the body and on the faces of women.
Terminal hair – This is the hair that is found on the scalp, arms, legs, pubic areas, ears and eyebrows and on the faces of men.

ACTIVITY

Try to describe a mutual friend or family member to another without mentioning the colour, length or shape of their hairstyle – how difficult is it?

Step 3
A horse-shoe section was made from the crown area to incorporate the side sections.

Step 4
The hair over the ear was cut without tension ensuring the overall length matches the lengths previously cut at the back.

Step 5
The fringe was cut using a freehand cutting technique.

Step 6
The haircut was cross-checked to ensure that the hair length on both sides of the cut matched each other.

145 · HAIRCUT: LEVEL 2 ONE LENGTH LOOK

Activity boxes Activity boxes provide additional tasks for you to complete to further your understanding of the unit. Some of them, if completed correctly, may even count towards your portfolio or key/core skills.

Step-by-step photographs Each cutting technique is illustrated by clear, colour, step-by-step photographs. The cutting techniques are clearly explained by the accompanying text. Some of the cutting techniques are also included as video clips on the CD-ROM. Look out for the CD-ROM symbols.

Tip boxes The author's experience is shared in the tip boxes. You will find plenty of positive suggestions to help you improve your knowledge and skills for each of the units and when working in the salon.

It's a fact! Your attention is drawn to some interesting and informative facts about the world of cutting hair.

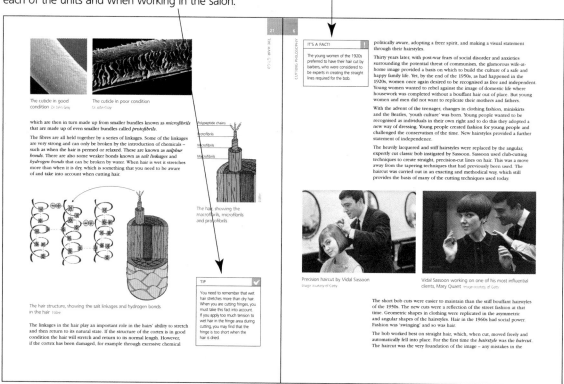

The cuticle in good condition Dr John Gray

The cuticle in poor condition Dr John Gray

which are then in turn made up from smaller bundles known as *microfibrils* that are made up of even smaller bundles called *protofibrils*.

The fibres are all held together by a series of linkages. Some of the linkages are very strong and can only be broken by the introduction of chemicals – such as when the hair is permed or relaxed. These are known as *sulphur bonds*. There are also some weaker bonds known as *salt linkages* and *hydrogen bonds* that can be broken by water. When hair is wet it stretches more than when it is dry, which is something that you need to be aware of and take into account when cutting hair.

Polypeptide chains

Protofibrils

Microfibrils

Macrofibrils

The hair, showing the macrofibrils, microfibrils and protofibrils

The hair structure, showing the salt linkages and hydrogen bonds in the hair

The linkages in the hair play an important role in the hairs' ability to stretch and then return to its natural state. If the structure of the cortex is in good condition the hair will stretch and return to its normal length. However, if the cortex has been damaged, for example through excessive chemical

TIP

You need to remember that wet hair stretches more than dry hair. When you are cutting fringes, you must take this fact into account. If you apply too much tension to wet hair in the fringe area during cutting, you may find that the fringe is too short when the hair is dried.

IT'S A FACT!

The young women of the 1920s preferred to have their hair cut by barbers, who were considered to be experts in creating the straight lines required for the bob.

politically aware, adopting a freer spirit, and making a visual statement through their hairstyles.

Thirty years later, with post-war fears of social disorder and anxieties surrounding the potential threat of communism, the glamorous wife-at-home image provided a basis on which to build the culture of a safe and happy family life. Yet, by the end of the 1950s, as had happened in the 1920s, women once again desired to be recognised as free and independent. Young women wanted to rebel against the image of domestic life where housework was completed without a bouffant hair out of place. But young women and men did not want to replicate their mothers and fathers.

With the advent of the teenager, changes in clothing fashion, miniskirts and the Beatles, 'youth culture' was born. Young people wanted to be recognised as individuals in their own right and to do this they adopted a new way of dressing. Young people created fashion for young people and challenged the conservatism of the time. New hairstyles provided a further statement of independence.

The heavily lacquered and stiff hairstyles were replaced by the angular, expertly cut classic bob instigated by Sassoon. Sassoon used club-cutting techniques to create straight, precision-cut lines on hair. This was a move away from the tapering techniques that had previously been used. The haircut was carried out in an exacting and methodical way, which still provides the basis of many of the cutting techniques used today.

Precision haircut by Vidal Sassoon
Image courtesy of Getty

Vidal Sassoon working on one of his most influential clients, Mary Quant Image courtesy of Getty

The short bob cuts were easier to maintain than the stiff bouffant hairstyles of the 1950s. The new cuts were a reflection of the street fashion at that time. Geometric shapes in clothing were replicated in the asymmetric and angular shapes of the hairstyles. Hair in the 1960s had social power. Fashion was 'swinging' and so was hair.

The bob worked best on straight hair, which, when cut, moved freely and automatically fell into place. For the first time the *hairstyle* was the *haircut*. The haircut was the very foundation of the image – any mistakes in the

Crossword and word searches These activities test the reader's retention of the information in the chapter.

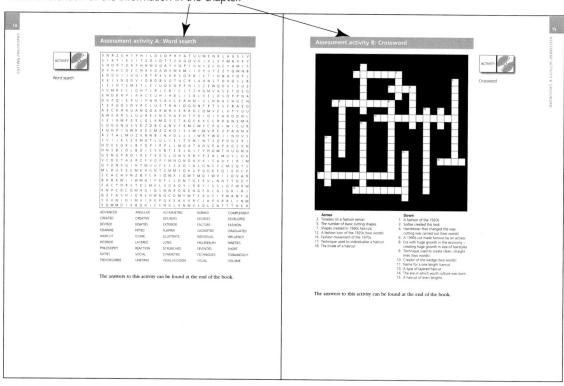

Assessment activity A: Word search

ACTIVITY

Word search

ADVANCED ANGULAR ASYMMETRIC BOBBED COMPLEMENT
CREATED CREATIVE DECADES DEGREES DEVELOPED
DEVISED EIGHTIES EXTERIOR FACTORS FASHION
FEMININE FIFTIES FLAPPER GEOMETRIC GRADUATED
HAIRCUT ICONIC ILLUSTRATE INDIVIDUAL INFLUENCE
INTERIOR LAYERED LONG MILLENNIUM NINETIES
PHILOSOPHY REACTION SCRUNCHED SEVENTIES SHORT
SIXTIES SOCIAL SYMMETRIC TECHNIQUES TONIANDGUY
TREVORSORBIE UNIFORM VIDALSASSOON VISUAL VOLUME

The answers to this activity can be found at the end of the book.

Assessment activity B: Crossword

ACTIVITY

Crossword

Across
2. Timeless (in a fashion sense)
5. The number of basic cutting shapes
7. Shapes created in 1960s haircuts
12. A fashion icon of the 1920s (two words)
16. Fashion movement of the 1970s
17. Technique used to individualise a haircut
18. The inside of a haircut

Down
1. A fashion of the 1920s
3. Sorbie created this look
4. Hairdresser that changed the way cutting was carried out (two words)
6. A 1990s cut made famous by an actress
8. Era with huge growth in the economy – creating huge growth in size of hairstyles (two words)
10. Creator of the wedge (two words)
11. Name for a one length haircut
13. A type of layered haircut
14. The era in which youth culture was born
15. A haircut of even lengths

The answers to this activity can be found at the end of the book.

Assessment of knowledge and understanding

All the activities at the end of each chapter relate directly to the knowledge and understanding that has been covered. The activities have been graded into different levels to suit individual readers, though it is always fun to try all the levels.

As a general guide:

Level A   This activity can be completed by those who are new to the industry and are following S/NVQ Level 2.

Level B   This activity can be completed by those who have completed S/NVQ Level 2 and are working towards Level 3.

Level C   These more challenging activities and be completed by those who are working towards S/NVQ Level 3 or higher qualification.

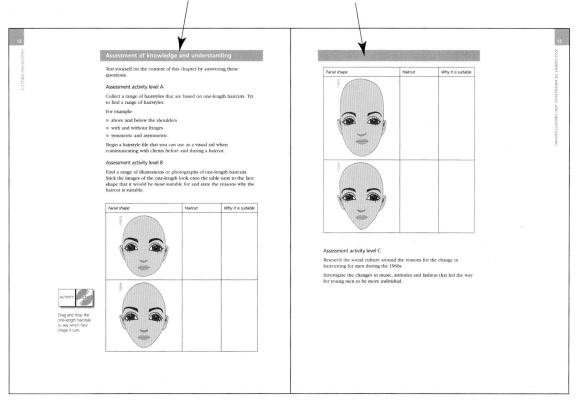

about the CD-ROM

A unique interactive learning CD-ROM accompanies *The Cutting Book*.
It allows you to step into a virtual salon and expand your cutting skills.
Key features of the CD-ROM include:

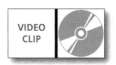

Video clips and step-by-steps

Video clips are provided to bring to life some of the cutting techniques
shown in the step-by-step photos in the book.

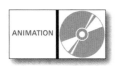

Animations and activities

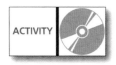

Animated diagrams and activities provide a practical demonstration of
various topics such as the science of the hair and skin.

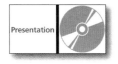

Presentations

Important information is broken down into bullet-point presentations of the
key facts.

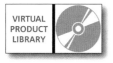

Virtual product library

A selection of styling and finishing products are stored in the virtual
product library allowing you to enhance your product knowledge
and to practice selecting everything you would need to carry out styling
and finishing.

'My Portfolio'

'My Portfolio' lets you save your work for your tutor or supervisor,
for future reference, or even to count towards your final assessment.

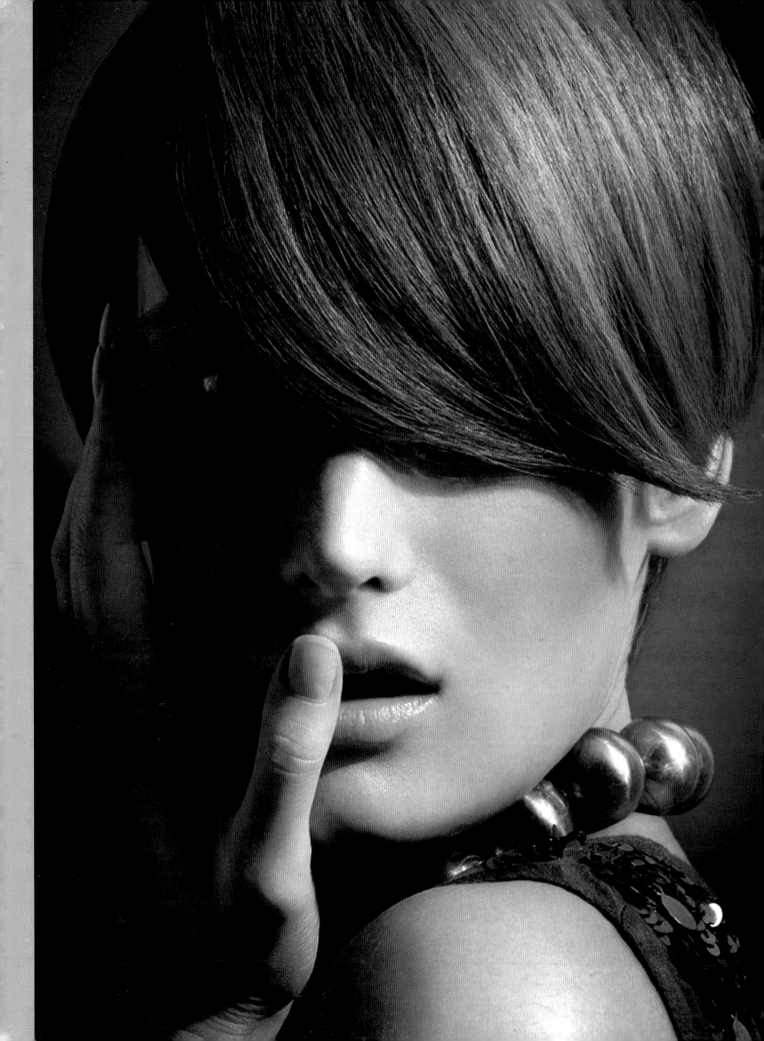

cutting philosophy

" The basic knowledge and foundation of a haircut is crucial. Without this grounding you can never create advanced cuts. So be patient with your learning and application. Get it right and then your creativity can expand and you can add other dimensions – creating individual aspects and a personal style statement. I believe a hairstyle is a continual journey. Each time you are faced with the same client you should approach their hair as if it is the first time you have cut it, relooking at what you have done, adding elements – for example additional layers – or use different products to get a slightly different result. Master this journey and your clients will remain faithful, because you are retaining your interest in them. Education and training should never stop. You can always improve your skills. "

ANTHONY MASCOLO

chapter 1

CUTTING PHILOSOPHY

Learning objectives

In this chapter you will learn about the social factors and philosophy that inspired iconic hairdressers from the last five decades to create haircuts that still have a major influence on the way haircutting is carried out today. You will see how the cutting techniques that were developed have been refined and adapted to create the new and exciting methods of cutting hair we now use.

To explore the extent of the influence of inspirational hairdressers and the techniques that they developed you will learn about:

- **how haircutting techniques have evolved to become the methods in use today**
- **how our individual image is formed by the hairstyle we wear**
- **how socio-economic factors influenced a range of haircuts of the last five decades**
- **how haircuts complement fashion**

INTRODUCTION

There are four basic cutting shapes that you will learn at the beginning of your hairdressing career. The shapes and the techniques you use to create them will provide the foundation on which more advanced techniques will be built.

The basic shapes are:

- one-length cut
- uniform layer
- short graduation
- long gradation.

ACTIVITY

Label the basic hair shapes

Once you have gained confidence and are competent at the four basic shapes, you can then build on these shapes to create a variety of looks using different cutting techniques. However, as you use the more advanced techniques, you will recognise that it is impossible to do these without first having a good basic shape on which to work.

Through this chapter you will see that the four basic cutting shapes are not new, nor are they unique to the twenty-first century, but they have been developed and have evolved over a period of time, particularly over the last 50 years. You will see that some aspects of the cutting you do today have been engineered and developed by creative and influential hairdressers who not only had individual ideas about how haircuts should be created, but also thought deeply about what the haircut represented in that particular period of time. This thought process can be described as *cutting philosophy*.

Cutting philosophy can also be described as the creative demonstration and interpretation of fashion. The creativity for some hairdressers is so imaginative that their influence goes far beyond the realms of one individual haircut. Their philosophy can last for decades.

HAIR CUTTING AND SOCIAL CULTURE, 1960 TO THE PRESENT

The word *culture* used in a social context can define how people are expected to behave in society. The rules determine how a person should think, feel, look and act. The rules may also include how a person should dress or style their hair.

Therefore, we can see that hairdressing as part of fashion, is sometimes used as a mechanism to demonstrate a reaction against what is expected. Sometimes, the wearing of particular hairstyles can be seen as a rebellion or revolution against mainstream society at any given time. At the same time, hairstyles can be used to perfectly complement the clothes and fashions of the time.

You may think that the developments in each fashion era are innovative and entirely new; yet it is easy to show that this is not the case and that someone has always been there before.

Influences for the one-length haircuts

When Vidal Sassoon created the geometric-shaped haircuts in the 1960s they were said to be the start of a new revolution in hairdressing. However, it is interesting to compare the philosophy behind the neat, clean lines of the 1960s with that of the bobbed hairstyles of the 1920s.

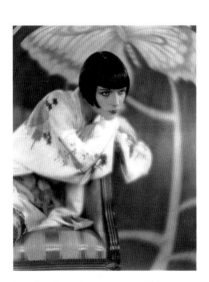

Louise Brooks, actress, 1921

The bobbed haircut of the iconic actress Louise Brooks in 1921, with its straight fringe and blunt edges, was a departure from the waves and soft feminine curls that preceded the 'flapper' fashion. The clean lines and easy-to-maintain bob hairstyle freed young women from the time-consuming efforts of maintaining their long hair. Women were beginning to be more

IT'S A FACT!

The young women of the 1920s preferred to have their hair cut by barbers, who were considered to be experts in creating the straight lines required for the bob.

politically aware, adopting a freer spirit, and making a visual statement through their hairstyles.

Thirty years later, with post-war fears of social disorder and anxieties surrounding the potential threat of communism, the glamorous wife-at-home image provided a basis on which to build the culture of a safe and happy family life. Yet, by the end of the 1950s, as had happened in the 1920s, women once again desired to be recognised as free and independent. Young women wanted to rebel against the image of domestic life where housework was completed without a bouffant hair out of place. But young women and men did not want to replicate their mothers and fathers.

With the advent of the teenager, changes in clothing fashion, miniskirts and the Beatles, 'youth culture' was born. Young people wanted to be recognised as individuals in their own right and to do this they adopted a new way of dressing. Young people created fashion for young people and challenged the conservatism of the time. New hairstyles provided a further statement of independence.

The heavily lacquered and stiff hairstyles were replaced by the angular, expertly cut classic bob instigated by Sassoon. Sassoon used club-cutting techniques to create straight, precision-cut lines on hair. This was a move away from the tapering techniques that had previously been used. The haircut was carried out in an exacting and methodical way, which still provides the basis of many of the cutting techniques used today.

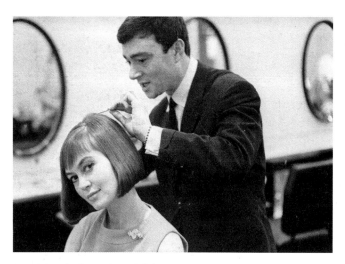

Precision haircut by Vidal Sassoon
Image courtesy of Getty

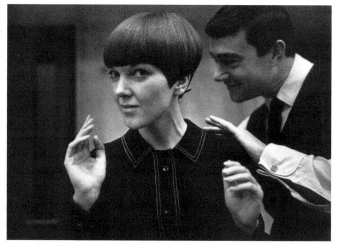

Vidal Sassoon working on one of his most influential clients, Mary Quant Image courtesy of Getty

The short bob cuts were easier to maintain than the stiff bouffant hairstyles of the 1950s. The new cuts were a reflection of the street fashion at that time. Geometric shapes in clothing were replicated in the asymmetric and angular shapes of the hairstyles. Hair in the 1960s had social power. Fashion was 'swinging' and so was hair.

The bob worked best on straight hair, which, when cut, moved freely and automatically fell into place. For the first time the *hairstyle* was the *haircut*. The haircut was the very foundation of the image – any mistakes in the haircut could not be disguised by styling. Therefore, the skill and art of haircutting took on new importance.

When you create your basic one-length cut you will see that the classic bob is still with us today. However, by clever use of creative texturising cutting techniques, the clean, exacting lines that define the classic image of the bob may be softened to complement the individuality of today's fashions.

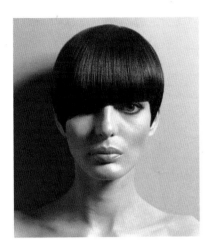 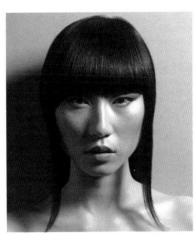

Hair: Gary Gill; make-up: Phyllis Cohen; photography: Paul Hopkins

Influences for layered haircuts

Following the relative prosperity of the post-war 1960s, the 1970s brought an economy in decline. Along with raging inflation came high unemployment and, for a short time, a three-day working week. Perhaps this is why the fashion for the decade seemed to be one of conflict.

Skirt lengths went from mini to midi to maxi, and on one side of fashion were romantically dressed girls in free flowing, floral dresses, yet on the other the beginnings of the punk movement. Punks were more aggressive in their desire to challenge the values of the existing society than the hippies of the 1960s. Their challenge, aggression and rebellion were particularly displayed through the hairstyles that have come to represent the punk era. Semi-shaven heads sporting brightly coloured Mohican spikes dominated punk images.

However, the punk look did not rely on expert cutting and was a contrast to another revolutionary haircut – the 'Wedge'.

Trevor Sorbie created the Wedge over 30 years ago, yet its design still forms the basis of the graduated haircuts you see today. This graduated haircut was defined by its short layers around the perimeter of the haircut that increased in length to the longer layers of the interior. The layers appeared to stack up on top of each other with each one so precisely cut that they gradually blended together to form the image that made Trevor Sorbie one of the most influential hairdressers of today.

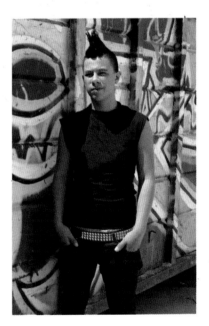

Punk hairstyles represent the anarchy of the 1970s

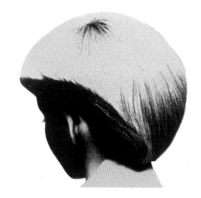

The precise cutting used for the Wedge ensures each layer blends together perfectly

The Wedge replicated some of the philosophies instigated by Vidal Sassoon – the clean lines, the precision cut and the shape of the haircut – that are still copied and frequently used in today's haircuts.

When you create your graduated cuts today you will use some of the very same techniques that Trevor Sorbie used to create his Wedge. Care must be taken with the angles that the hair is held. Short graduation occurs when the hair is held and cut at between 45° and 90° from the scalp. The angles are critical for the amount of graduation found in the final result. You will read about the effects and use of angles in haircutting in Chapter 5, Cutting Techniques.

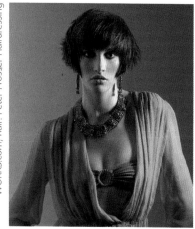

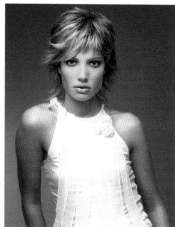

Photographer: Paul Hopkins www.THE-IMAGE-WORKS.com; hair: Peter Prosser Hairdressing

Hair: Vicky Turner for Goldsworthy's; photographer: Martin Evening; clothes styling: Tracy Goldsworthy; make-up: Janet Francis

Contemporary interpretations of graduation

A short graduated haircut is best carried out on hair that is straight, though variations can also be seen as graduated haircuts on hair that is wavy or curly.

The layered haircuts that were first created in the 1970s were cut with the same precision as those of the previous decade. However, by the 1980s, hair was becoming big.

This expansion in the size of hair can be illustrated if we compare a layered cut designed by the Toni & Guy Artistic Team in 1977, which is expertly cut and blow-dried, with the layered, 'scrunched' look designed by Trevor Sorbie in 1980, where the amount of volume in the hair in a similarly shaped and length-layered haircut has been increased by the use of scrunch-drying and products.

The big, often curly hair of the 1980s reflected the change in fashion and social attitudes. The recessions of the 1970s were over and there was a surge in growth of the economy, with people spending more on themselves than ever before. Society was consumerism-based and greed was seen as something to strive for. Women in particular made an authoritative statement with their clothing through the use of shoulder pads. 'Power dressing' became the norm for working women, who often wore masculine trouser suits. Thus, the wide hair complemented the wide shoulders and the curls softened the masculine look to the clothing. In the 1980s even *short* hair was big! The graduated haircuts, which previously would have lain on the head in the exact way they had been cut, were root dried to increase volume.

Layered haircuts today can still have a 1980s feel, with volume and lift at the roots, exaggerating the look of the basic cut. Once again this demonstrates how haircuts that were designed over 20 years ago still have an influence on the styling and cutting techniques we use today. This is because the hairdressers who designed the cutting techniques were inventive and forward-thinking.

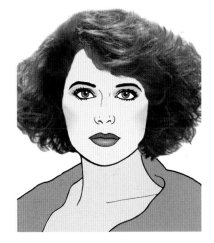

Layered hair is scrunched to create volume

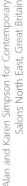

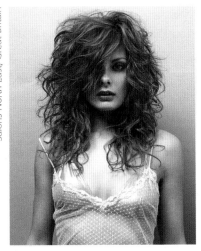

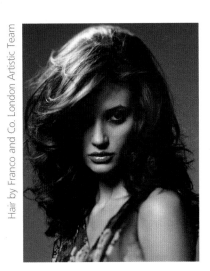

Alan and Karen Simpson for Contemporary Salons North East, Great Britain

Hair by Franco and Co. London Artistic Team

Contemporary cuts with a 1980s feel for lift and volume

This forward thinking can be demonstrated by the early techniques used for texturising. Today we use a wide range of freehand cutting methods to texturise the hair to create individual designs tailored to each client's own hair length, texture and type. However, Sassoon-type club-cutting techniques were widely used until the early 1980s, when some hairdressers began experimenting and there was a move away from the precise cutting techniques. Edges began to be softened and in more extreme examples, the whole look was shattered by cutting into the haircut in an apparently random, but calculated way. Trevor Sorbie's 'Chop' was the forerunner of the freehand texturising techniques you can use today.

While curly hair was dominant in the 1980s, and into the early 1990s, by the middle 1990s, straight hair once again became fashionable. The change in look had a great deal to do with the change in fashion. From the excesses

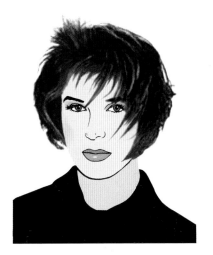

The Chop, by Trevor Sorbie, introduced the concept of texturising

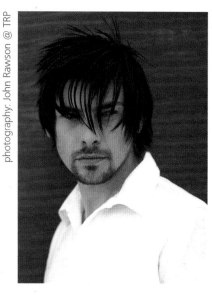

Hair: the Anne McGuigan Art Team, Leighton Buzzard; photography: John Rawson @ TRP

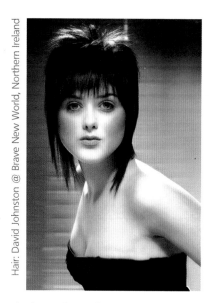

Hair: David Johnston @ Brave New World, Northern Ireland

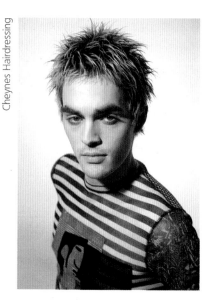

Cheynes Hairdressing

Texturised looks created by using similar techniques introduced over 20 years ago

of the 1980s came a more minimalist look, where less was more. Clothes became neat and more tailored – out went the wide shoulder pads and in came sleek silhouettes; bright brash colour changed to muted tones of grey or black, chunky knits to fine and glitter to shimmer.

The two major haircut shapes of the 1990s were the long graduated layer and the chunky uniform layer. Both haircuts were created for and worn by two actresses and became the most asked-for haircuts in history. The long graduated 'Rachel' cut and the short layered cut worn by Meg Ryan once again demonstrated the need for highly skilled precise cutting techniques that had evolved over the previous four decades.

The long, graduated Rachel cut was created by having longer texturised layers on the perimeter of the haircut and shorter layers on the interior, often including a 'grown-out' fringe.

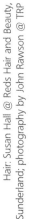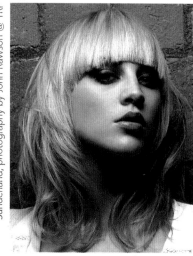

Hair: Susan Hall @ Reds Hair and Beauty, Sunderland; photography by John Rawson @ TRP

Graduated haircuts with shorter layers extending to longer layers on the exterior of the haircut

For shorter hair, the chunky but texturised layered looks were based on a classic uniform layer haircut. Holding the hair at right angles (90°) to the scalp creates the uniform layers. However, the use of individualised slicing, chopping, pointing and chipping techniques, plus a range of hairstyling products, gave the layered look much more movement and interest.

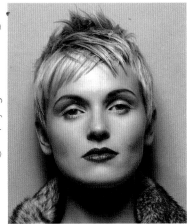

Hair: Keith Hall Creative Team; photography: John Rawson @ TRP; make-up: Liz Rochford @ TRP; styling: Karen Russell @ TRP

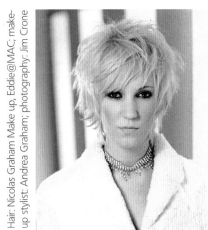

Hair: Nicolas Graham Make up, Eddie@MAC; make-up stylist: Andrea Graham; photography: Jim Crone

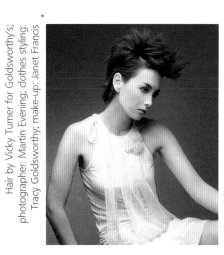

Hair by Vicky Turner for Goldsworthy's; photographer: Martin Evening; clothes styling: Tracy Goldsworthy; make-up: Janet Francis

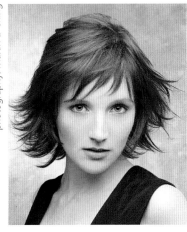

Hair: Bruno Miarli, Altered Image; photography: Martin Evening

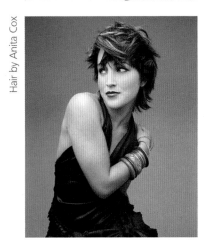

Hair by Anita Cox

Contemporary cuts showing chunky texturised looks

In the new millennium, it can be seen that cutting techniques and fashions of the previous five decades have come full circle. Sassoon used his cutting techniques to create a look that did not rely on 'hair dressing'. The same can be said of today's looks. The accuracy of the haircut is the most important requirement of current hair fashions. Hairdressers are not relying on styling techniques to create the image. Instead, by simply using the shape and movement created during the haircut, the hairstyle is formed.

Therefore, whether you are taking your first tentative steps for haircutting, experimenting and developing your more creative techniques, or refining and perfecting your cutting as an experienced hairdresser, you can do two things. First, look back through recent history to gain inspiration from iconic hairdressers – then look forward, think creatively and experiment bravely.

Assessment of knowledge and understanding

Test yourself on the content of this chapter by answering these questions.

Assessment activity level A

Collect a range of hairstyles that are based on one-length haircuts. Try to find a range of hairstyles.

For example:

- above and below the shoulders
- with and without fringes
- symmetric and asymmetric.

Begin a hairstyle file that you can use as a visual aid when communicating with clients before and during a haircut.

Assessment activity level B

Find a range of illustrations or photographs of one-length haircuts. Stick the images of the one-length look onto the table next to the face shape that it would be most suitable for and state the reasons why the haircut is suitable.

Facial shape	Haircut	Why it is suitable
Habia		
Habia		

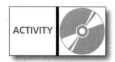

Drag and drop the one-length hairstyle to see which face shape it suits

Facial shape	Haircut	Why it is suitable
Habia		
Habia		

Assessment activity level C

Research the social culture around the reasons for the change in haircutting for men during the 1960s.

Investigate the changes in music, attitudes and fashion that led the way for young men to be more individual.

Assessment activity A: Word search

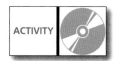

Word search

```
V N R Z G H T P H I L O S O P H Y A T U U M E N R L A U S I V
S I X T I E S I T E O J D T T Z V G Q V K J X L V F M A V F Y
S H O R T D A F H N W U G A Y V G P J G N S Z C G C Y H M I S
D V H H C D E C N A V D A W E M X M I I D P U Y Z Z Y G M N B
E D G U I J O G J R T R E V O R S O R B I E T I O N A Y Q F L
V E I S N Q D V I O B D B V G T U C R I A H N S T O X G J L B
I S J O T E M E T L E J U O E O P F H I S Z E W Q O V I S U Z
S U M R E C L O H T L R J C B I C J T Z H Q M V A S E T D E G
E N D B R P J A A C E U H I H B L I S B L X E L O S O P P N A
D G P Q I E P U I P N N S A V C E R N M I V L N N A C H G C N
T Z F U O S D Y P C I U S T R H I D G O N T P T S S F B A E G
A E C K R A U A N Q O A R W R V E R R D C Q M V E L X T Y U U
B W E A R S L U U R E S N C P A E H T P O I O I E A O O D N L
S E I G W F E E L Q L K M G S S T A Q E K X C C R D B N E M A
C O G U N U S V K Z D B C U N V F E M C M Y C P G I W I C U R
F Q H P I G W K E E C M Z Z H O I S S W I M V R E V P A A N X
R S T A L M U Z V N N B I N V D L J J I W R Y W D J I N D V S
S V I J K S Z E M Q T L U L S E I T E N I N T S Q P O D E R J
H O E E G K L B Y D P I R P L L M G A T A O V E A P K G S X N
H N S B I O L B O I S S E B T E E J G J T Y H O M T H U G N X
G E N U P R O I R E T X E S L O N V R B Y P Z H L M U Y L O K
V C D E T A E R C F V Q P F M N Q N D A X X I S A U Y J K I M
G Y D N X G I H T W U U F E E Z X O I A L G N S Y C M S Q T S
M L D U E Z C M K H G N T S M M Y O K U P G D K E Q I E H C P
S C A C H V N Z B Y C R I Q W X I G W T M D I W V I J O V A R
B K B K W I I W M N I F O F L L D N T O E E V L N H T T G E Y
F A C T O R S T E C M K L V O A Q Y I R B Y I S S L O F W R W
K N P C D C O M A G I Q S W W R O G E N G F D L G I G K I R J
Q Z F A S H I O N E H W N Q C D M Y W T E A U Y I P W A N F G
Y E V N I D I M V J R E P Q X E A V V R C J A P U R R L I N M
E Q M M D J X B O H I C C N G L V N W V S Q L Z N T T T H E H
```

ADVANCED	ANGULAR	ASYMMETRIC	BOBBED	COMPLEMENT
CREATED	CREATIVE	DECADES	DEGREES	DEVELOPED
DEVISED	EIGHTIES	EXTERIOR	FACTORS	FASHION
FEMININE	FIFTIES	FLAPPER	GEOMETRIC	GRADUATED
HAIRCUT	ICONIC	ILLUSTRATE	INDIVIDUAL	INFLUENCE
INTERIOR	LAYERED	LONG	MILLENNIUM	NINETIES
PHILOSOPHY	REACTION	SCRUNCHED	SEVENTIES	SHORT
SIXTIES	SOCIAL	SYMMETRIC	TECHNIQUES	TONIANDGUY
TREVORSORBIE	UNIFORM	VIDALSASSOON	VISUAL	VOLUME

The answers to this activity can be found at the end of the book.

Assessment activity B: Crossword

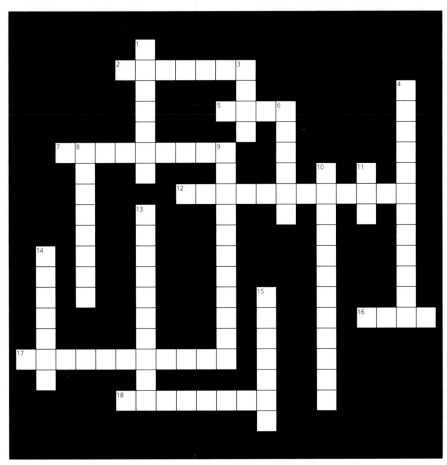

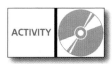

Crossword

Across
2. Timeless (in a fashion sense)
5. The number of basic cutting shapes
7. Shapes created in 1960s haircuts
12. A fashion icon of the 1920s (two words)
16. Fashion movement of the 1970s
17. Technique used to individualise a haircut
18. The inside of a haircut

Down
1. A fashion of the 1920s
3. Sorbie created this look
4. Hairdresser that changed the way cutting was carried out (two words)
6. A 1990s cut made famous by an actress
8. Era with huge growth in the economy – creating huge growth in size of hairstyles
9. Technique used to create clean, straight lines (two words)
10. Creator of the wedge (two words)
11. Name for a one length haircut
13. A type of layered haircut
14. The era in which youth culture was born
15. A haircut of even lengths

The answers to this activity can be found at the end of the book.

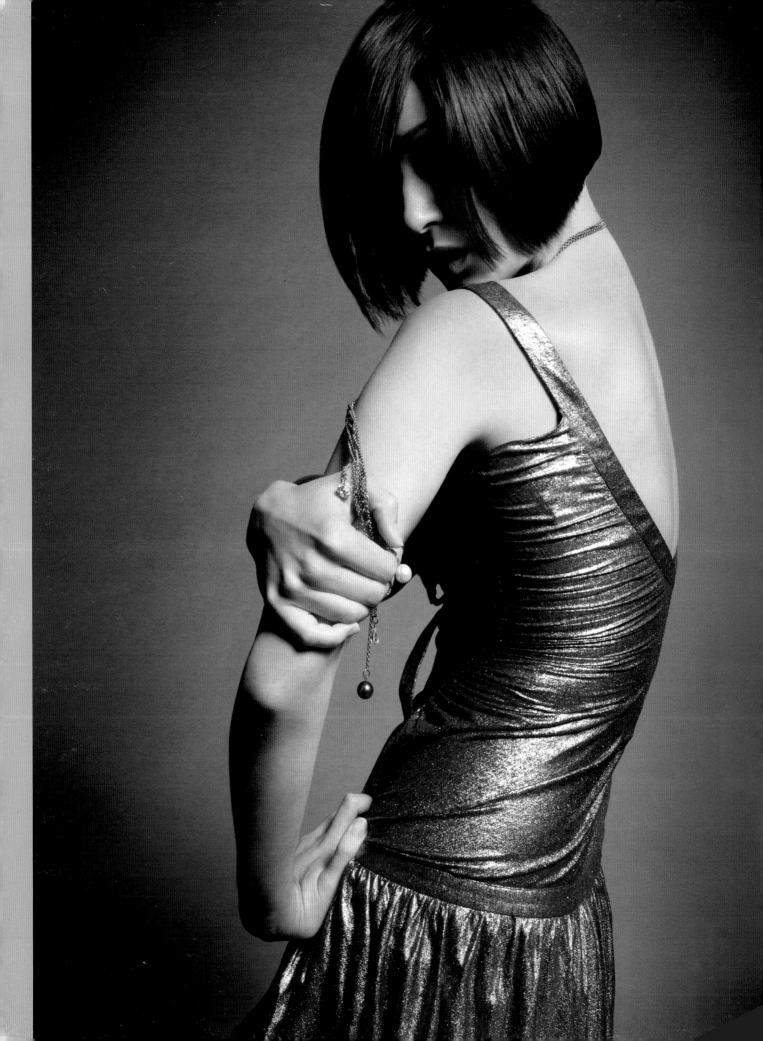

hair and skin structure and analysis

" It is vital that to satisfy any client's needs, and to carry out your work in a professional capacity, a full hair and scalp analysis is conducted. Scalp and hair health, condition, sensitivity levels, porosity and general condition are all crucial to both hair and colouring services from a technical aspect. Understanding your client's hair in terms of texture, condition, density and type is crucial to ascertaining how their hair will behave and assessing their hair's capabilities correctly. Home care advice is also part of our team's consultation process. Skin tone, face shape and eye colour are all essential to prescribing the right cut or colour and giving the client the overall look they want; and in keeping them happy you can ensure they will become repeat business. "

RICHARD WARD, RICHARD WARD HAIR & METROSPA, LONDON

chapter 2

HAIR AND SKIN STRUCTURE AND ANALYSIS

Learning objectives

In this chapter you will learn about the structure and characteristics of the hair within the skin. This is a critical area of learning for cutting hair. The way you cut hair will depend on every aspect of hair structure and hair growth analysis. If you fail to conduct an extensive consultation with your client, you will not have the necessary information to perform a successful haircut – and your client will leave dissatisfied. Therefore, you need to learn about the different hair types, textures and growth patterns, and how cutting techniques are adapted and used. In addition, you need to know how hair density influences the way you cut hair and how the properties of elasticity in the hair can determine the way in which you cut it. In order to recommend a suitable look for the client, you must be able to identify the shape of the client's head. Therefore, you will also learn about the face bones and muscles of the head and face.

In this chapter you will learn about:

- **the structure of the hair and skin**
- **the hair growth cycle**
- **hair growth patterns**
- **factors affecting hair growth**
- **hair type**
- **hair texture**
- **hair density**
- **hair elasticity**
- **changes in the hair structure that affect styling and finishing**
- **bones and muscles of the head and face**

This chapter links to the following S/NVQ units

G7 Advise and consult with clients

G9 Provide hairdressing consultation services

INTRODUCTION

The construction of the hair and skin is a fascinating subject. Hair covers the majority of our bodies and the skin is our largest organ. Yet sometimes we can take it all for granted – we just expect it to be there. However, as hairdressers and barbers, we have to know and understand how the characteristics of the hair and skin affect the hairdressing and barbering services, and, in particular, haircutting.

Before you can begin to cut your client's hair, you must be able to analyse the structure and characteristics of the hair and skin. Each and every client will be unique and your consultation results will reflect this.

THE STRUCTURE OF THE HAIR AND SKIN

The hair on our heads is one of the most distinctive things about us. When you describe one person to another, you probably describe their hair and hairstyle before you talk about the features of their face such as the colour of their eyes.

Our hair varies in length, style and colour, and even the diameter of each individual strand. With your hair you can make statements about yourself. You can say – 'I am outrageous', or 'I am shy and reserved'. You can look very professional, or you can choose to look unkempt. You can have a haircut that looks fashionable or you can have a look that is timeless and classic.

ACTIVITY

Try to describe a mutual friend or family member to another without mentioning the colour, length or shape of their hairstyle – how difficult is it?

THE HAIR

Hair grows all over the body, except on the soles of the feet, the palms of the hands and the eyelids. However, some types of hair have different characteristics to other types.

There are three types of human hair:

Lanugo hair – This type of hair is soft and downy and found on newborn babies. This hair is lost soon after birth.

Vellus hair – This is the fine hair that is found all over the body and on the faces of women.

Terminal hair – This is the hair that is found on the scalp, arms, legs, pubic areas, ears and eyebrows and on the faces of men.

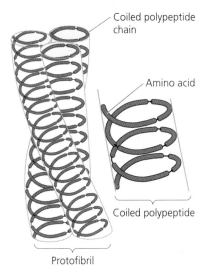

Coiled polypeptide chain

Amino acid

Coiled polypeptide

Protofibril

Cross-links within the hair

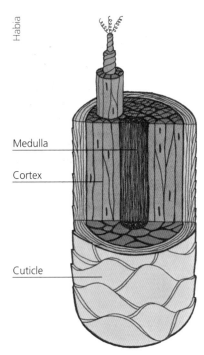

Medulla

Cortex

Cuticle

Hair structure in cross-section

The chemical structure of hair

Hair has the same keratin structure as nails, horns, claws, feathers and fur. The main structure of the hair, the bundles of the *cortex*, is made up from molecules of amino acids. *Amino acids* are the basic structural building units of proteins. They form short chains called *peptides* or *polypeptides*, which in turn form into the protein *keratin*. There are 22 amino acids in the hair, which contain elements of carbon, hydrogen, nitrogen, oxygen and sulphur.

The structure of hair

Hair is made up of three sections. They are:

- the cuticle
- the cortex
- the medulla.

Cuticle

The cuticle is the outermost part of the hair. It is made up of overlapping layers of translucent scales. The scales are sometimes likened to tiles of a roof in the way that each lies over the other. The scales of the cuticle play an important part in the condition of the hair. Hair that is in good condition will have a cuticle that lies flat and is smooth. A smooth cuticle makes it easier to brush and comb the hair and reflects the light to give a glossy appearance. If the cuticle is damaged the uneven or broken cuticle layers make the hair tangle easily and because the cuticle does not lie flat and smooth light does not reflect from it, making the hair look dull.

There are a number of reasons why the cuticle may be damaged. It can be damaged from over-processing with chemicals, from brushing, combing and using heated appliances without correctly protecting the hair with products, or from tying the hair into unsuitable bands. Alternatively, the hair may be damaged by the environment, for example, suffering from excessive sun and wind damage. You can find out how good the condition of the cuticle is by carrying out a porosity test. The method for carrying out this test is found in Chapter 3, The Art of Consultation and Communication.

The number of layers of the cuticle is one of the factors that determine the texture of hair. Hair that is fine will be smaller in diameter and have fewer layers of cuticle than hair that is coarse.

Cortex

The cortex is the main section of hair and it is within this section that the properties of elasticity and strength exist and where the chemical changes for colouring, bleaching, perming and relaxing processes occur. The cortex is made up of intertwining, coiled bundles of elongated, cigar-shaped cells that twist together. The bundles within the cortex are called *macrofibrils*,

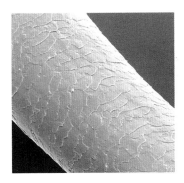

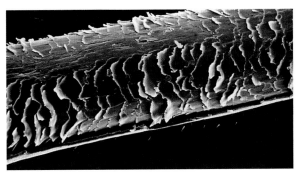

The cuticle in good
condition Dr John Gray

The cuticle in poor condition
Dr John Gray

which are then in turn made up from smaller bundles known as *microfibrils* that are made up of even smaller bundles called *protofibrils*.

The fibres are all held together by a series of linkages. Some of the linkages are very strong and can only be broken by the introduction of chemicals – such as when the hair is permed or relaxed. These are known as *sulphur bonds*. There are also some weaker bonds known as *salt linkages* and *hydrogen bonds* that can be broken by water. When hair is wet it stretches more than when it is dry, which is something that you need to be aware of and take into account when cutting hair.

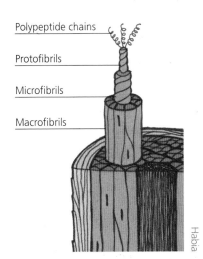

The hair, showing the
macrofibrils, microfibrils
and protofibrils

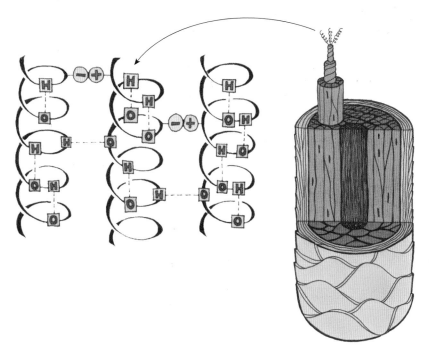

The hair structure, showing the salt linkages and hydrogen bonds
in the hair Habia

The linkages in the hair play an important role in the hairs' ability to stretch and then return to its natural state. If the structure of the cortex is in good condition the hair will stretch and return to its normal length. However, if the cortex has been damaged, for example through excessive chemical

TIP ✓
You need to remember that wet hair stretches more than dry hair. When you are cutting fringes, you must take this fact into account. If you apply too much tension to wet hair in the fringe area during cutting, you may find that the fringe is too short when the hair is dried.

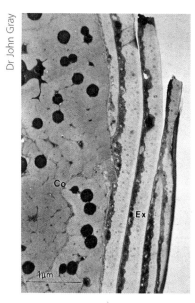

Dr John Gray

Cross-section of hair showing granules of keratin in the cortex

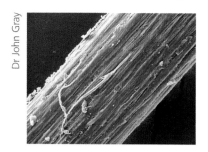

Dr John Gray

Cross-section of hair exposing bundles of cortical cells

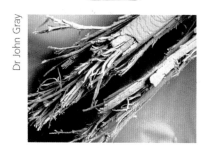

Dr John Gray

Badly damaged hair revealing damage to the cortex

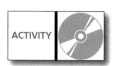

ACTIVITY

Identify whether the hair is in good or bad condition

treatments, the hair will break under tension, or remain in a stretched state. You can find out how good the elasticity is in the hair by carrying out an elasticity test. The method for carrying out this test is found in Chapter 3, The Art of Consultation and Communication on p. 57.

The colour pigment *melanin* is also found within the cortex. The natural and artificial colours of hair can be seen through the translucent cuticle cells.

Medulla

The medulla is a space that may be found within the central core of coarse hair. Fine hair may not have a medulla. However, as the medulla is only made up of soft spongy cells with air spaces and has no function, it does not matter if it is present or not.

ACTIVITY

Look at the photographs of the hair structure and determine whether the hair is in good or poor condition.

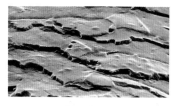

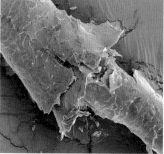

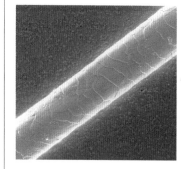

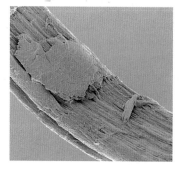

Identify the condition of the cuticle and cortex Dr John Gray

---

THE SKIN

The hair is situated within the skin, which is actually the largest organ of the body. The skin comprises of two main layers – the *epidermis* and the *dermis*. The dermis is the layer in which all the appendages of the hair are found.

Epidermis

The epidermis is the outer layer of the skin, which is made up of the dead skin cells that are constantly being rubbed away or shed. Excess shedding of dead skin cells on the scalp can be seen as dandruff. There are five layers (or strata) of the epidermis, and each one has different characteristics.

The five layers are:

1 stratum corneum
2 stratum lucidum
3 stratum granulosum
4 stratum spinosum
5 stratum germiniativum.

> **IT'S A FACT** !
>
> The word 'stratum' means 'layer'.

- **Stratum corneum** – In this layer, the skin cells are flat and resemble scales. The dead cells are rubbed off by friction, and if not removed they form dry patches of scale on the skin surface, making it look dry and dull.

- **Stratum lucidum** – These cells do not have a nucleus and are clear in appearance. At the bottom of this layer is a fatty substance which prevents the absorption of liquids into the body.

- **Stratum granulosum** – Within this layer the transition occurs from living to dead cells. *Keratinisation* takes place within this layer, which is the hardening of the skin cells. Excessive keratinisation can lead to the skin condition *psoriasis*.

- **Stratum spinosum** – This layer is also known as the prickle cell layer due to the appearance of the cells, which have fine, spiky projections. Chemical changes in this layer lead to the eventual keratinisation which makes the skin hard and durable.

- **Stratum germinativum** – In this layer the cells are constantly dividing by a process known as *mitosis*. The cells then gradually make their way through the other layers of the epidermis until they die and are shed from the surface of the skin. The pigment melanin is found in this layer.

> **IT'S A FACT!** !
>
> Mitosis is the division of cell nuclei where one cell splits into two, then two become four, four become eight and so on.

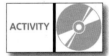

ACTIVITY

Label the five layer of the epidermis

> **IT'S A FACT!** !
>
> Between 70 and 90 per cent of the dust in a house is made up of dead skin cells that have been shed from the body. It is on these skin cells that dust mites feed.

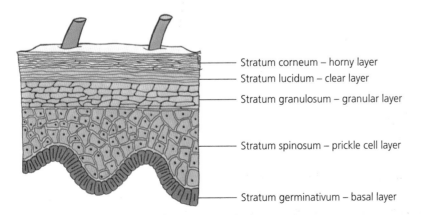

Stratum corneum – horny layer
Stratum lucidum – clear layer
Stratum granulosum – granular layer
Stratum spinosum – prickle cell layer
Stratum germinativum – basal layer

The five layers of the epidermis Habia

Dermis

The dermis is also known as the 'true skin', and it is within this section that the appendages to the hair and the blood and nerve supply are found.

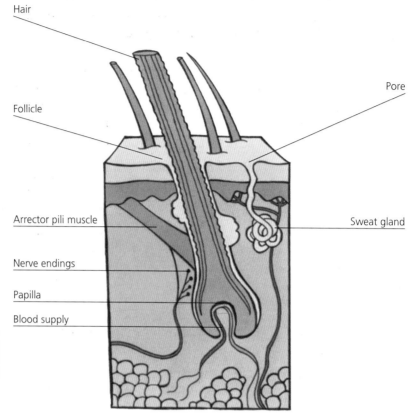

Cross-section of the skin Habia

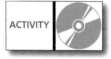

Label the cross-section of the skin

- **Follicle** – All the follicles you have are developed before birth and are a tubular down growth in the dermis that holds and supports the hair in place. Follicles vary in size, depending on the type of hair that grows from it. For example, a follicle containing a vellus hair will be smaller than one that contains a terminal hair.

- **Sebaceous gland** – This is the gland that produces the natural oil of the hair and scalp called *sebum*. Sebum lubricates the hair to provide gloss to the hair and protection to the skin. Clients with an underactive sebaceous gland are likely to have hair that is dry in condition and it may look dull. However, if the sebaceous gland is overactive, too much sebum will be produced and the client will have oily hair.

- **Sweat gland** – The sweat gland is also known as the *sudoriferous gland*. This produces sweat which is made up of water, salts and other minerals. The release of sweat through the sweat duct onto the skin is used as a mechanism to cool the skin when you get hot. The cooling effect occurs when the moisture on the skin is evaporated.

- **Arrector pili muscle** – This is a muscle that works involuntarily. This means that you are not able to control the muscle yourself. If you get cold or frightened, the muscle will contract of its own accord and make the hair stand up. When the muscle is contracted the effect it has on the skin is known as 'goose pimples'. At the same time that you get goose pimples, the hair (depending on its length) will stand on end, or be raised. This action helps you to either trap warm air if you are cold or act as a warning system if you are frightened. An extreme action of the arrector pili muscle can be seen on cats or dogs who, when alarmed, raise their fur to make them look larger and more aggressive as a form of protection.

- **Nerve endings** – The hair does not have its own nervous system, and therefore you cannot feel when the hair shaft has been cut. But the follicle itself is surrounded by a network of nerves which enables you to feel any movement in the hair. In addition, the dermis contains a variety of nerve endings or *receptors*. Each one of the nerve endings is specially designed to detect different sensations, which occur on the skin. For example, some are designed to detect changes in temperature, while others enable you to feel pain. Pressure nerve endings can also be found in the dermis as well as those that can detect the lightest touch of the skin.

- **Blood supply** – The hair itself does not have a blood supply – if it did, it would bleed when the hair was cut. However, the blood supply is very important, as it carries nutrients that ensure healthy hair growth. The blood supply enters the dermal papilla through a series of fine small blood capillaries. The dermal papilla is the point from which all new cells for hair growth are produced. As well as supplying nutrients required for the development of new growth, the blood supply helps to remove waste products.

- **Papilla** – This is the point at which all new cells for hair growth are produced. When first formed, the cells produced are very soft, but they are hardened (keratinised) and shaped as they are forced into the follicle and out onto the surface of the skin.

The functions of the skin

The functions of the skin are:

- protection
- absorption
- excretion and secretion
- temperature control
- sense of touch.

Protection

The skin is known as the largest organ of the body and one of its functions is to protect other organs within the body. It does this by creating a barrier around the body which prevents the invasion of micro-organisms. In addition to the skin itself, another line of defence to micro-organisms is the *acid mantle*. The acid mantle is a protective layer that is made up of a combination of sweat and sebum, which ensures that the pH of the skin

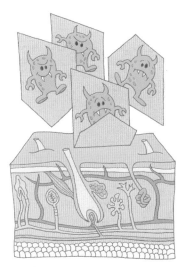

Skin function of protection

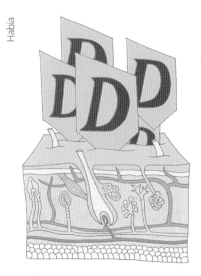

Habia

Skin function of absorption

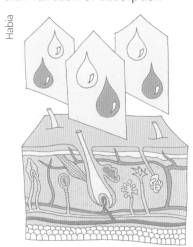

Habia

Skin function of excretion and secretion

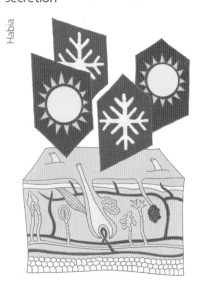

Habia

Skin function of temperature control

is maintained at around 4.5–5.5. The skin is also able to detect danger. It does this via the nerve endings, which can track extremes of heat and cold as well as pain from something that may penetrate the surface of the skin, thus protecting the body from harm.

Absorption

While the skin acts as a barrier and prevents harmful micro-organisms entering the body, it is capable of a limited amount of absorption. The skin absorbs Vitamin D, which is derived from sunlight. Vitamin D is essential for the body as it aids the formation of healthy bones.

Excretion and secretion

The skin excretes sweat, which helps to dispose of excess salts in the body as well as helping to cool the skin when you are too warm. Another excretion is that of the natural oil of the skin – sebum. Sebum helps to moisturise the skin and hair in order to prevent excessive dryness.

Temperature control

The organs of the body are designed to work at our normal body temperature of 36.8°C or 98.6°F, so it is important that this temperature is maintained. If you are too hot or too cold, your body can adjust the temperature in two main ways – one through the blood supply and the other by the production of sweat. If you get too hot the sudoriferous (sweat) glands produce sweat, which then evaporates from the skin surface, producing a cooling effect. In addition to this, the blood vessels expand – making you look pink or sometimes very red – again allowing your temperature to be reduced. If you are too cold, the blood vessels contract making you look pale, and, in extreme cases, you can look very blue. By doing this, the blood vessels are reducing the amount of heat that is lost by the body. In addition to this, the muscles of the body can involuntary contract, causing you to shiver. This action helps to keep you warm. The arrector pili muscle is linked to control of body temperature. When you are cold, the arrector pili muscle contracts, creating goose pimples and causing the hair to stand up. This effect can be clearly seen on the arms, where the hair is short. The air trapped in the hairs helps to retain body heat.

Sense of touch

The dermis contains many sensory nerve endings which can transmit messages to the brain to ensure that you are aware of your surroundings. Some nerve endings allow you to detect the most minute and delicate touch, others tell you if something is hot or cold, and those that lie deeper within the dermis detect pressure or tension. Sometimes the sense of touch can be clearly defined and used as a means of communication. For example, when cutting hair you need to make direct contact with your client during the consultation. This type of touch is known as *physical communication* and is very important in gaining your client's trust and confidence. For example, during the consultation you may hold the client's hair with your hands to illustrate how you will cut the hair, to show the client the potential length of the haircut. You will read more about physical communication in Chapter 3, The Art of Consultation and Communication.

ACTIVITY

You can see the effects of touch by touching the skin on the back of the hand or the arm with a metal, two-pronged roller or hairpin. First, bend the ends of the roller or hairpin and separate them so they are 5 cm apart. Then, working with a partner, ask them to close their eyes while you touch different areas on the back of their hand or arm. Ask your partner how many points they can feel on their skin – one or two? You will discover that areas of the skin with more nerve receptors will allow you to feel two points. Where there are fewer nerve receptors, you will only feel one point – even though two have been used.

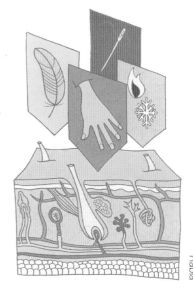

Skin function of sense of touch

HAIR GROWTH CYCLE

The hair on our head grows, falls out and grows again in a continual cycle of time that can last anything from 1.5 to 7 years. Hair grows at an average rate of 1.25 cm each month. If the cycle is disrupted, the hair may fall out and not be replaced. When this happens, the distribution of hair becomes sparser; in some cases bald patches will appear.

There are three main stages to the hair growth cycle. They are known as:

- anagen
- catagen
- telogen.

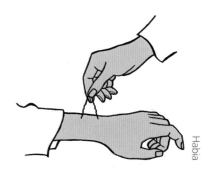

Experiment to illustrate the sense of touch

Anagen

Have you ever wondered why some people have very long hair, while others struggle to achieve a length that reaches past their shoulders? This variation in the ability to grow hair is due to the active growing stage of the hair, a stage which is known as *anagen*. It can last from around 1.5 years to up to 7 years. Those people who have an active anagen stage of 7 years can grow their hair to a longer length than those with an anagen stage of only 1.5 years. During the anagen stage the hair is constantly fed by the blood supply to the dermal papilla, where the colour of the hair is determined as well as the texture and type.

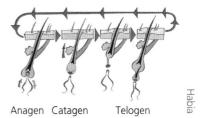

Anagen   Catagen   Telogen

The three stages of hair growth

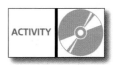

Label the three stages of hair growth

Catagen

This stage is relatively short in length – it only lasts for around two weeks. During this stage the follicle rests and new cell production ceases at the dermal papilla. The follicle begins to detach itself from the blood supply and begins to shrink away from the dermal papilla.

Telogen

This stage can be described as the complete resting stage of hair growth. At this point the follicle completely separates from the papilla for a period of around four months. At the end of the resting stage, the follicle re-attaches itself to the papilla and the blood supply once again supplies the nutrients to allow new hair growth, starting a new anagen stage. If the follicle failed to reattach itself to the papilla, the new anagen stage would not begin and the client would experience hair loss, such as alopecia or as in male pattern baldness.

HAIR GROWTH PATTERNS

The haircut and eventual hairstyle will be, in part, determined by the direction of hair growth. The direction of hair growth will be unique to every client and should be identified at the consultation stage. There are three main areas that you need to check prior to beginning a haircut. They are the:

- front hairline
- crown area
- nape area.

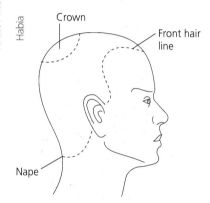

Habia

Areas of adverse hair growth patterns

Front hairline growth patterns

Some clients' hair will grow straight down at the front hairline. This means that there are no adverse hair growth patterns. Therefore, you can cut a fringe in such a client's hair and when the hair is styled it will lie in the position that it has been cut. However, other clients have hair that grows in a few or many different directions, which means that the hair growth pattern may prevent them from having a fringe that lies flat to the head.

Adverse front hairline growth patterns

The two main adverse hair growth patterns found at the front hairline are known as:

- cowlick
- widow's peak.

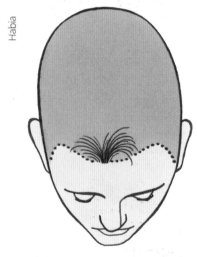

Habia

Cowlick

Cowlick A cowlick is frequently found on one or both sides of the forehead hairline. The hair generally grows back from the hairline meaning that the hair will stick up if a short fringe is cut. However, having a cowlick can be an advantage if you wish to create a fringe that is spiky and requires lift in the fringe area. Some cowlicks vary in extreme more than others. Some merely have a slight change in direction of hair growth, while in others the hair grows straight back across the entire front hairline.

Widow's peak With this type of hair growth pattern, the hair initially grows back from a deep point at the centre of the forehead. Alternatively, the hair on both sides of the centre of the forehead may grow into the middle to form a point. The growth pattern is usually symmetrical, at the centre of the forehead, and because of this it is very difficult to cut a fringe into the hairstyle.

Crown hair growth patterns

The crown is generally the area at the top of the head. At this point you can quite clearly see the circular growth pattern of the hair. The vast majority of clients only have one crown, but some have a double crown where you will be able to see two clear areas of circular growth. Sometimes the two crowns are very separate, but the two crowns may overlap, creating an area of hair that grows in many different directions, ultimately making it difficult to control and style if it is cut too short.

On some clients the 'crown' or circular area of growth is not at the top of the head in the place you may expect it, but is on the side, or lower down towards the occipital bone. For these clients you must ensure that the growth pattern will not adversely affect the final look of the haircut.

Nape hair growth patterns

Clients who do not have adverse hair growth patterns at the nape area will have hair that will lie flat or neatly at the nape – even when it is cut very short. However, most clients have hair that grows in one, two or even more different directions at the nape of the neck.

The swirling patterns of hair are known as *nape whorls* and they can be seen on one or both sides of the neck. Sometimes the nape whorls grow in the same direction. For example, the hair may grow from the left to the right. On other clients you may see the hair growing from the right to the left. However, sometimes the hair grows in opposite directions on either side of the centre of the nape area, which means that the hair then grows into a tail of hair at the centre.

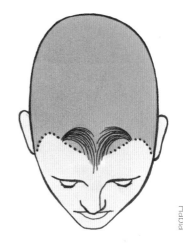

Widow's peak

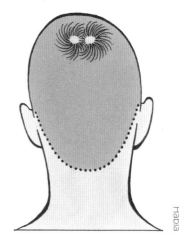

Double crown

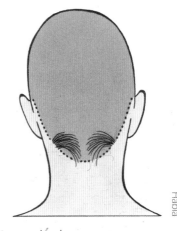

Nape whorls

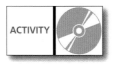

Identify the hair growth patterns

IT'S A FACT!	!

If you look at the head of a baby when their hair first starts to grow you can quite clearly see all the different growth pattern directions. You will be able to see the circular pattern at the crown and swirls at the nape and front hairline.

TIP	✔

Avoid haircuts and cutting techniques that will cause a problem with the variety of different hair growth directions. Work with the hair growth instead of fighting against it. For example, a client whose hair grows towards the centre at the nape of the neck can easily wear a hairstyle where the nape area is cut into a V shape.

FACTORS AFFECTING HAIR GROWTH

Following a haircut you must make a recommendation to the client about when their hair should be cut again, in order for them to maintain the condition or the look of their hair. Some client will have hair that grows at different rates to others. There are several factors for this. They are:

- **Ethnic origin** – Some hair types appear to grow more quickly than others. The sleek straight hair of Asian origin does grow more quickly than African-type hair, but the apparent slowness in growth is partly because African-type hair has a tendency to curl tightly at the roots.

- **Hereditary** – Male pattern baldness is hereditary, which means that if your male client's father or grandfather (on either the mother's or father's side of the family) had hair loss, your client is likely to have a similar pattern of baldness.

- **Medication** – Some types of drugs can inhibit or slow down hair growth – or in some cases, as with chemotherapy, cause the hair to fall out. However, there are some drugs – for example, steroids – that cause excessive hair growth in unwanted places – such as on faces of women.

- **Length of hair growth cycle** – Some clients have a longer anagen stage than others, thus they will be able to grow their hair for a longer period of time.

- **Diet** – A healthy balanced diet is essential for healthy hair growth. Protein is particularly important, as is iron. Drastic crash dieting can lead to hair loss.

- **Hormones** – Changes in hormone levels are thought to be one of the causes of alopecia. In menopausal women, changes in hormone levels can also lead to hair loss.

Hair type

The way you cut the hair and the technique you use will depend on the correct analysis of the features and characteristics of your client's hair type. You need to be able to determine the amount of curl, wave or straightness in the hair before you begin the haircut.

Hair type refers to how straight, how wavy or how curly the hair is. The hair, curl, wave or straightness can be natural or it can be chemically induced. For example, a client may have naturally curly hair, but they may have straightened it with chemical – therefore, the structure and appearance of the hair will have changed. Likewise, the client may have naturally straight hair, but may have had a perm to increase the amount of body and movement in the hair. The change in the natural state of the hair can also be temporary. For example, if curly hair is stretched when it is dried, it can look straight.

Ascertaining hair type is one reason why you need to talk to your client about their hair when conducting the hair analysis. If you do this, and recognise the true hair type – i.e., how curly, wavy or straight the hair is – you will be able to make the correct decisions about which cutting technique to use, and be able to correctly advise the client about the final, finished result.

You must ensure that you conduct the hair analysis to determine the type of hair when the hair is dry and when it is wet. Curly or wavy hair can appear to be straight when it is wet and may give you a false impression of the characteristics of the hair.

The type of hair your client has is not only down to the direct generic inheritance from their parents, but is also a great deal to do with their ancestors.

Hair can be classified into three generic types:

- African
- Caucasian or European
- Asian.

African-type hair

African-type hair is sometimes known as African Caribbean hair. However, it is important to recognise that this type of hair is not restricted to those people who have originated from the Caribbean. African-type hair is generally very curly, and often frizzy, but the type of curl can vary from soft, open curls to tight, woolly hair. This type of hair is found not only on people of African decent, but also on people of mixed race. Sometimes, hair with similar characteristics to African type hair – tight, frizzy curls – can be seen on a client who is obviously Caucasian. African-type hair is generally dark in colour; it is frequently brown, dark brown or black, but can also be red or blonde. Sometimes, African-type hair may seem as though it does not grow as quickly as Asian or Caucasian hair, which is true to some extent. However, as the hair is very crinkled, it grows in a variety of directions before it appears to gain length. In addition to this, although the hair may look coarse, it is often very fine and delicate, meaning that it is likely to break before reaching a great length. Therefore, you have to treat this hair very gently when combing and brushing.

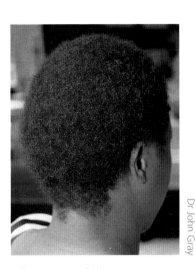

African-type hair

Dr John Gray

TIP	✔
The best technique for cutting very tightly curled hair into an 'Afro' shape is to comb the hair into shape and then cut the outline with long-bladed scissors or with clippers.	

The types of cutting techniques that can be used for African-type hair are:

- **Club-cutting** – This can be used on hair that is natural or chemically treated hair that has been relaxed or permed.
- **Freehand cutting** – Once combed into place, African-type hair stays in place, so freehand cutting is much easier to carry out.
- **Clipper cutting** – Clippers can be used to reduce the length and to create lines and shapes in natural African-type hair. Because the hair stays in place the clippers can glide easily across the surface. The clippers can also be used over a comb to create graduated looks.

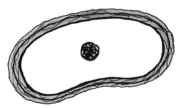

Cross-section of African-type hair

Habia

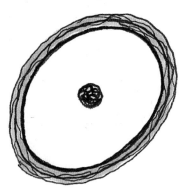

Cross-section of Caucasian hair Habia

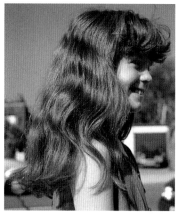

Caucasian-type hair Dr John Gray

Caucasian- or European-type hair

Caucasian or European hair has very many different characteristics. This type of hair can be straight, wavy or curly, coarse or fine in texture, and may vary in colour from black to the palest blonde. The differences in Caucasian hair in Britain are the result of people from all over Europe and beyond invading or inhabiting the British Isles for hundreds of years. Blonde, straight Caucasian hair is attributed to the Viking people who invaded Britain in 878 AD. Red, sometimes coarser, hair can be linked to the Celts from Scotland, who were in turn invaded or occupied by five different ethnic groups during the Dark Ages. Dark brown glossy hair can be linked to the Romans who ruled in Britain from 43 AD, while dark curly hair can be linked with the Roma Gypsies who lived in Britain at the same time. Thus Caucasian hair is never the same from one client to another. It can be coarse and curly or fine and straight, it can have the characteristics of African-type hair or those more associated with Asian hair. Therefore, you really need to carry out a very careful analysis of your client's hair before you begin to carry out a haircutting service.

The best techniques for cutting Caucasian hair will vary depending on the characteristics of your client's hair. However, remember that club-cutting will retain the bulk and reduce the length in hair, whereas texturising will reduce both the length and bulk in hair. Tapering hair, which leaves finer ends, will increase the amount of curl and movement in the hair, so you may wish to avoid using this technique on clients with curly hair.

Asian-type hair

Asian hair includes the dark glossy hair that you associate with India or Pakistan, and the much straighter, Oriental-type hair found in the Far East – China and Japan. While Japanese hair is very straight, there may be some limited wave and movement in other types of Asian hair. Asian hair is normally very dark brown or black in colour. This type of hair grows much faster than Caucasian or African-type hair and is often much coarser.

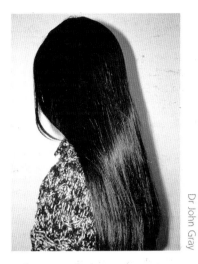

Dr John Gray

Asian-type hair

> **TIP** ✓
>
> Slicing and deep pointing techniques work particularly well on hair that is strong and straight. You also need to pay close attention to the hair growth patterns at the nape and crown as the strength and structure of the hair can make it very difficult to style when cut short.

> **IT'S A FACT!** !
>
> If you look at Asian hair under the microscope you will see that the cross-section of the hair is round.

You need to be aware that it is unlikely that your clients have the exact characteristics of the three generic hair types described. This is because, over many thousands of years, the different hair types have been mixed up – leading to a sort of melting pot of hair types. This is one reason why the types of cutting you will use are individualised to meet the exact requirements of each client's own hair type and characteristics.

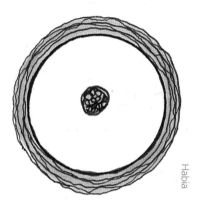

Habia

Cross-section of Asian hair

> **IT'S A FACT!** !
>
> Asian hair grows out of the scalp at an almost perpendicular angle.

Hair texture

Hair can be divided into three main divisions and then subdivided again. The three main categories for hair texture are:

- coarse
- medium
- fine.

The categories can be further subdivided into the following categories:

- very coarse to coarse
- coarse to medium
- medium to fine
- fine to very fine.

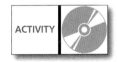

ACTIVITY

Identify the cross sections of hair

Coarse hair

One of the characteristics of coarse hair is that it quite often feels dry. Clients with coarse hair normally have fewer hairs per square centimetre than clients with fine hair. An average head of hair has 100,000 individual

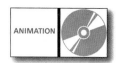

Layers of cuticle

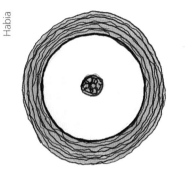

Coarse-textured hair may have up to 11 layers of cuticle

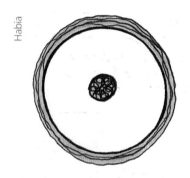

Fine-textured hair may only have four layers of cuticle

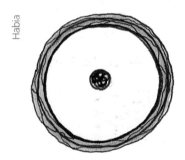

Medium-textured hair, with seven layers of cuticle

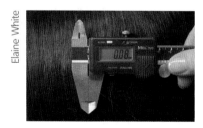

Vernier callipers measuring a single strand of hair

strands. Fine-haired clients can have as many as 150,000 hairs, while clients with coarse hair may only have 80,000. Therefore, some clients with coarse hair may also have sparse hair and clients with fine hair may have an abundance of hair.

The physical appearance of the diameter of coarse hair is larger than that of a fine hair and may have up to 11 layers of overlapping cuticle layers and coarse hair normally has a medulla.

Fine hair

Fine hair may only have four layers of overlapping cuticle layers and as a result may be much more liable to damage and breakage. The medulla is often missing in fine hair – though as the medulla serves no purpose in hairdressing terms, this does not really matter. It is often assumed that fine hair is also sparse, though it is equally possible that it is abundant.

Medium hair

In terms of characteristics, medium hair falls between coarse and fine hair. It normally has around seven layers of cuticle. The medulla in medium hair can appear and then disappear, though this does not have any effect on the haircut or the properties of the hair.

Each of the hair textures reacts differently to the different cutting techniques. For example, fine hair can look thicker if club-cutting techniques are used. Texturising can add movement and interest to all textures of hair, though you would need to be careful with the amount of texturising you use in very fine hair, especially if it is sparse, to ensure that you do not remove too much weight.

An instrument known as a *micrometer* can measure the diameter of a single hair. The hair is placed within the anvil and spindle of the micrometer and its size is measured in microns. A *micron* is one millionth of a metre. Fine hair has a diameter of less than 50 microns, whereas the diameter of very coarse hair is around 120 microns. The diameter of hair can also be measured by *Vernier callipers*, which give a much easier-to-read, digital measurement.

ACTIVITY

Obtain a micrometer or set of digital Vernier callipers and see if you can take some measurements of hair. It is interesting to note that the hair will vary in texture on one head. You will find that on a head of very fine hair, you will also find some hair that is much coarser.

Hair density

Hair can be described as being *dense* (or abundant) or it can be *sparse*. If hair is abundant, it means that a client will have a greater number of hairs on their scalp than clients with sparse hair.

The texture, type and colour of hair can be directly related to density. The human scalp is approximately 770 square centimetres in size, and research carried out by Drs Erasmus Wilson, Withof and Stelwagon found the following:

- Caucasian blonde hair is the most abundant type of hair with around 146,000 hairs.
- Black hair is sparser, with a density of 110,000 hairs.
- Densities of red hair were between 86,000 and 100,000 hairs.
- The density of African-type hair is between 50,000 and 110,000 hairs.
- Asian hair has densities of between 80,000 and 140,000 hairs.

Some sparseness of hair can be isolated to particular areas of the scalp. It is common for men and women to have sparse areas at the temples. Male pattern baldness can affect the crown area, and, for some women hair may also be thinner on the top of the head from the frontal area to the crown.

Male pattern baldness

Male pattern baldness is probably the most noticeable aspect of hair density on your male clients. This is a genetically inherited condition. If the client's father or grandfather had hair loss through male pattern baldness, then he too is likely to have a similar condition.

The most common pattern of male pattern baldness is known as the *Hamilton Pattern*.

In the Hamilton Pattern you can see that the hair thins first at the temporal area and then the crown. The hair then becomes sparser across the top of the head until the areas of baldness merge together, leaving only the hair at the sides and back of the head. The time that this hair loss takes will vary from client to client, from a few to many years.

Alopecia

Sparse hair can also be attributed to alopecia. No one really knows what causes alopecia, but the most common reasons connected to hair loss through alopecia are stress and changes in hormone levels. However, whatever the causes, the results can be devastating for clients.

The term *alopecia* covers a variety of conditions. *Alopecia areata* means that the hair loss occurs in circular or oval patches which can be seen on any area of the head.

If the alopecia areata condition continues, the bald patches can join together and eventually lead to a condition known as *alopecia totalis*, which means that there may be hair loss over the whole of the scalp.

During the consultation prior to cutting hair, you must check for areas of sparseness or hair loss. This is particularly important with male clients who may have grown their hair longer in some places in an attempt to disguise the hair loss. The client may not be happy if you cut off too much hair from these areas.

IT'S A FACT!

Male pattern baldness can be inherited from the mother as well as the father.

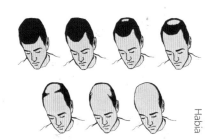

Hamilton Pattern baldness

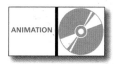

Hamilton pattern baldness

IT'S A FACT!

Alopecia areata can occur anywhere on the body. Areas of hair loss can be seen on arms and legs and even on the eyebrows.

HAIR ELASTICITY

The properties of elasticity in the hair allow you to temporarily change the look and structure of your hair. The ability of the hair to stretch and return to its original length depends on the structure and condition of the cortex. Within the cortex are a series of linkages (or bonds) that lie horizontally and vertically between the cortical cells. Some of the bonds, the sulphur bonds, are very strong and can only be broken by chemicals that are used to permanently curl or straighten the hair. However, water or applied, gentle heat can temporarily break the other bonds, the salt linkages and hydrogen bonds.

It is the weaker bonds that provide the opportunity for you to style and change the look of your client's hair. This temporary change in the hair structure will last until either the hair is wet again, or it has absorbed moisture from the atmosphere. When this happens, the bonds in the hair will revert to their original position and hairstyle.

You need to be aware of the hair's ability to stretch when you are cutting hair. When hair is wet, it stretches more than when it is dry. This is because the hydrogen bonds and salt linkages within the cortex are temporarily broken. So, if you cut hair wet, be aware that the hair will look shorter when you have dried it. This is especially important when you are cutting the fringe area or if there is any curl or wave movement in the hair.

CHANGES IN THE HAIR STRUCTURE THAT AFFECT STYLING AND FINISHING

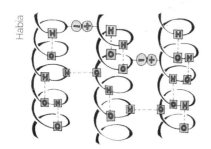

Sulphur, salt and hydrogen bonds found in the cortex of the hair

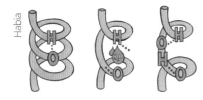

The change from alpha to beta keratin

The properties in hair that allow the shape to be temporarily changed during the styling and finishing of a haircut are directly related to the formation and structure of bonds within the cortex. There are three different types of bond. They are:

- sulphur bonds
- salt bonds
- hydrogen bonds.

Chemicals such as perm lotion can only break the sulphur bonds, but the salt and hydrogen bonds are weaker and are broken by water, atmospheric conditions and gentle heat. This means that the hair can be stretched and shaped into a new temporary position.

When hair is in its natural state, the formation of keratin is called *alpha keratin*. When the hair has been stretched and dried, the keratin formation is known as *beta keratin*. The new position remains in place until the bonds are broken again by water or moisture in the atmosphere. When this happens, the hair goes back to its natural state and the formation of the keratin is once again known as alpha keratin.

THE BONES AND MUSCLES OF THE HEAD AND FACE

The bones and muscles of the head and face determine the shape of the head and face and the features that your client has. Therefore, it is important to know the position of the bones and muscles.

The bones of the head and face

The skull is made up of bones that form the cranium and the face. The *cranium* encloses and protects the brain. In total there are 22 bones in the skull. Eight of the bones form the cranium and there are fourteen bones in the face. Seven of these facial bones determine the shape of the face. The remaining seven form the deeper facial cavities.

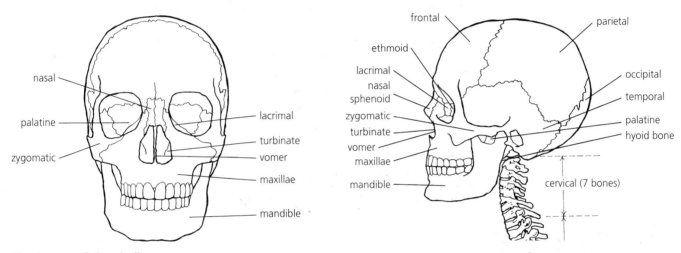

The bones of the skull Habia

While the position and proportion of all the bones of the skull determine the overall shape of your client's head and face, there are some bones that have more of a visual influence than others. For example, the shape of the occipital bone can make the back of the head look very round or very flat and you may have to create a look that enhances or disguises extremes in the size of the occipital bone. The height of the frontal bone will determine the shape and the length of fringe you cut for a client. The position and prominence of the zygomatic bone will determine the appearance of your client's cheekbones. And the shape of the mandible will determine the appearance and shape of the jawline.

The muscles of the head and face

The muscles, which lie over the bones, provide the shape and contours of the head and face. Some muscles can contract to allow movement, for example, the opening and closing of the mouth or eyes. Other muscles create movement and expression on the face – as when smiling or frowning. When muscles are toned, the contours of the face will be firm, but when the tone is lost, the muscles will sag, changing the appearance of the face – as can be seen during the course of the the ageing process.

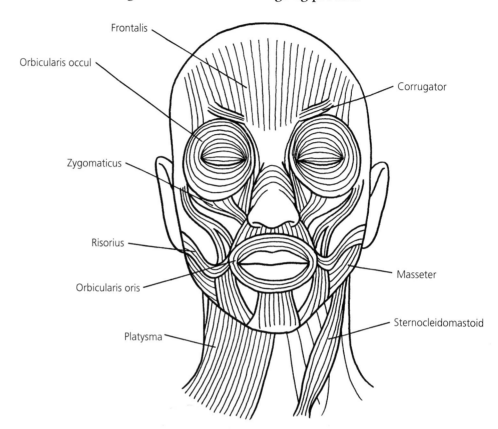

The muscles of face and head Habia

Assessment of knowledge and understanding

Test yourself on the content of this chapter by answering these questions.

Assessment activity level A

Label the skin diagram.

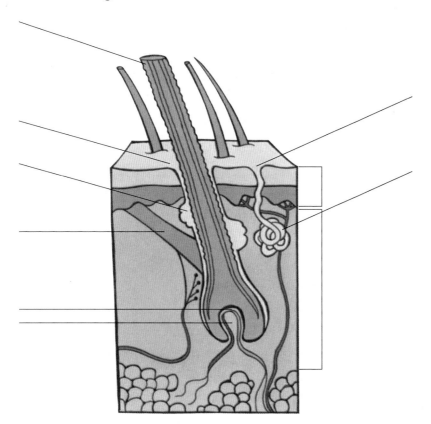

Habia

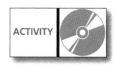

Label the skin
diagram

Label the hair diagram.

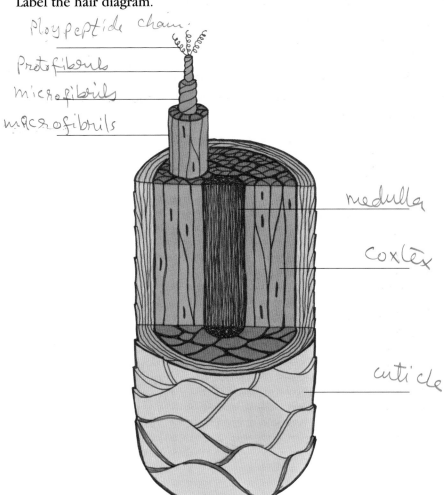

Ploypeptide chain

Protofibrils

microfibrils

macrofibrils

medulla

coxtex

cuticle

Habia

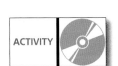

ACTIVITY

Label the hair
diagram

ACTIVITY

Multiple-choice
questions

Assessment activity level B

Select the correct answers:

1 Hair grows all over the body except the
    a hands
    b feet
    c eyelids
    d head

2 The soft downy hair that is found growing on the faces of women is
    known as
    a vellus hair
    b terminal hair
    c lanugo hair
    d soft hair

3 The outermost section of the hair is known as the

  a cortex
  b cuticle
  c medulla
  d melanin

4 The section of hair that contains the bonds responsible for the elasticity of the hair is the

  a cortex
  b cuticle
  c medulla
  d melanin

5 The skin is able to absorb

  a vitamin A
  b vitamin B
  c vitamin C
  d vitamin D

6 The arrector pili muscle allows

  a sebum to be formed
  b the hair to grow
  c the hair to remain in the follicle
  d the hair to stand on end

7 The uppermost layer of the epidermis is the stratum

  a germinativum
  b spinosum
  c corneum
  d lucidum

8 The natural oil of the hair and skin is

  a grease
  b sebum
  c oil
  d serum

9 Telogen is the

  a resting stage of the hair growth cycle
  b growing stage of the hair growth cycle
  c active stage of the hair growth cycle
  d stopping stage of the hair growth cycle

10 Curly hair is categorised as a

  a density
  b style
  c texture
  d type

The answers to this activity can be found at the end of the book.

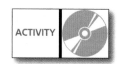

ACTIVITY

The bones of the
head and face

Assessment activity level B

Look at the diagram of the bones of the head and face and identify the
following:

- frontal bone
- occipital bone
- mandible
- zygomatic bone

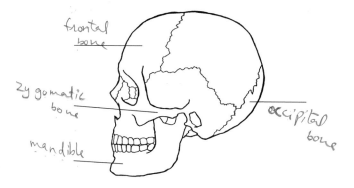

The answers to this activity can be found at the end of the book.

Assessment activity level C

1 Describe the cuticle section of hair.
2 List the five layers of the epidermis.
3 List the functions of the skin.
4 Describe the three stages of hair growth.
5 Describe the main characteristics of the three generic types of hair.

The answers to this activity can be found at the end of the book.

Assessment activity level A: Word search

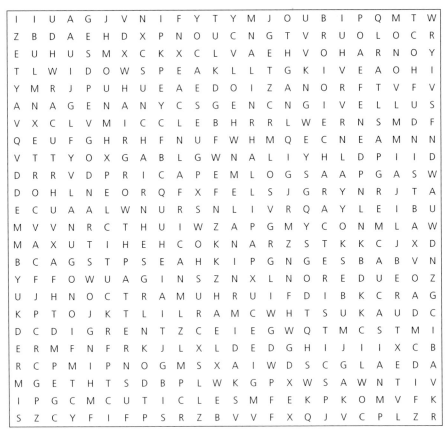

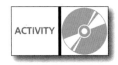

Word search

I	I	U	A	G	J	V	N	I	F	Y	T	Y	M	J	O	U	B	I	P	Q	M	T	W
Z	B	D	A	E	H	D	X	P	N	O	U	C	N	G	T	V	R	U	O	L	O	C	R
E	U	H	U	S	M	X	C	K	X	C	L	V	A	E	H	V	O	H	A	R	N	O	Y
T	L	W	I	D	O	W	S	P	E	A	K	L	L	T	G	K	I	V	E	A	O	H	I
Y	M	R	J	P	U	H	U	E	A	E	D	O	I	Z	A	N	O	R	F	T	V	F	V
A	N	A	G	E	N	A	N	Y	C	S	G	E	N	C	N	G	I	V	E	L	L	U	S
V	X	C	L	V	M	I	C	C	L	E	B	H	R	R	L	W	E	R	N	S	M	D	F
Q	E	U	F	G	H	R	H	F	N	U	F	W	H	M	Q	E	C	N	E	A	M	N	N
V	T	T	Y	O	X	G	A	B	L	G	W	N	A	L	I	Y	H	L	D	P	I	I	D
D	R	R	V	D	P	R	I	C	A	P	E	M	L	O	G	S	A	A	P	G	A	S	W
D	O	H	L	N	E	O	R	Q	F	X	F	E	L	S	J	G	R	Y	N	R	J	T	A
E	C	U	A	A	L	W	N	U	R	S	N	L	I	V	R	Q	A	Y	L	E	I	B	U
M	V	V	N	R	C	T	H	U	I	W	Z	A	P	G	M	Y	C	O	N	M	L	A	W
M	A	X	U	T	I	H	E	H	C	O	K	N	A	R	Z	S	T	K	K	C	J	X	D
B	C	A	G	S	T	P	S	E	A	H	K	I	P	G	N	G	E	S	B	A	B	V	N
Y	F	F	O	W	U	A	G	I	N	S	Z	N	X	L	N	O	R	E	D	U	E	O	Z
U	J	H	N	O	C	T	R	A	M	U	H	R	U	I	F	D	I	B	K	C	R	A	G
K	P	T	O	J	K	T	L	I	L	R	A	M	C	W	H	T	S	U	K	A	U	D	C
D	C	D	I	G	R	E	N	T	Z	C	E	I	E	G	W	Q	T	M	C	S	T	M	I
E	R	M	F	N	F	R	K	J	L	X	L	D	E	D	G	H	I	J	I	I	X	C	B
R	C	P	M	I	P	N	O	G	M	S	X	A	I	W	D	S	C	G	L	A	E	D	A
M	G	E	T	H	T	S	D	B	P	L	W	K	G	P	X	W	S	A	W	N	T	I	V
I	P	G	C	M	C	U	T	I	C	L	E	S	M	F	E	K	P	K	O	M	V	F	K
S	Z	C	Y	F	I	F	P	S	R	Z	B	V	V	F	X	Q	J	V	C	P	L	Z	R

HAIR
CHARACTERISTICS
COLOUR
CORTEX
CUTICLE
SEBUM
CATAGEN
PAPILLA
CAUCASIAN
AFRICAN
SLICING
WIDOWSPEAK
ANAGEN
EPIDERMIS
VELLUS

LANUGO
STRAND
TEXTURE
FOLLICLE
DERMIS
MELANIN
HAIRGROWTHPATTERNS
TELOGEN
ASIAN
TAPERING
CLUB
COWLICK
DERMIS
CUTICLE

The answers to this activity can be found at the end of the book.

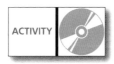

ACTIVITY

Crossword

Assessment activity level B and C: Crossword

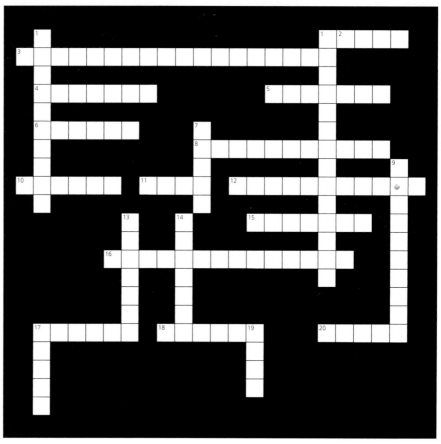

Across
2. Moisturises the skin and hair
3. Makes the hair stand up (three words)
4. Complete resting stage of the hair
5. Colour pigment
6. Which hair texture may have up to 11 cuticle layers?
8. Absorbs moisture
10. Main section in the hair
11. Number of layers in the epidermis
12. Carries nutrients to the hair (two words)
15. Not always present in the hair structure
16. The way the hair lies (two words)
17. Active growing stage of the hair
18. The 'true skin'
20. Hair type

Down
1. Function of the skin
2. Produces natural oil (two words)
7. Number of stages in the hair growth cycle
9. To stretch and return to its original length
13. The cross-section of which type of hair is kidney shaped?
14. Like tile on a roof
17. Hair classification
19. Largest organ in the body

The answers to this activity can be found at the end of the book.

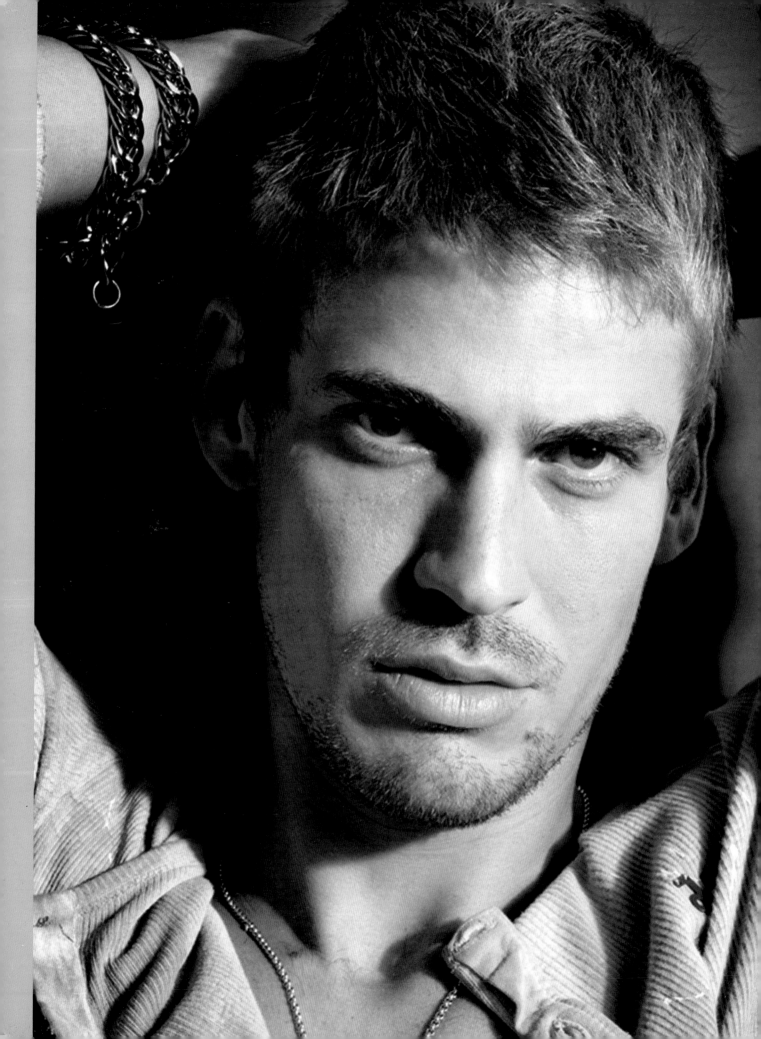

the art of consultation and communication

We all know that good hairdressing is 50 per cent communication and 50 per cent skill. It is crucial that each client receives a professional, full consultation. NEVER shampoo a client without giving them a proper consultation. It is the most essential part of our job! That five extra minutes spent on a detailed consultation would alleviate 99 per cent of customer complaints/dissatisfaction!

The key is to always ask open questions, such as 'how', 'why', 'tell me', 'where', 'what', and not closed questions which will automatically give short answers such as 'no', 'yes', 'don't know!'

When people leave their hairdresser, these are the top three reasons they normally give:

1 They always did what *they* wanted to do.
2 They didn't listen to me or suggest anything new.
3 They did something too drastic.

So, take this into account, think about how you communicate with your clients and you will know what not to do. Bear in mind that price concerns are hardly ever the reason that clients do not return!

HELLEN WARD, MANAGING DIRECTOR OF THE RICHARD WARD HAIR & METROSPA

chapter 3

THE ART OF CONSULTATION AND COMMUNICATION

Learning objectives

In this chapter, you will gain the skills you need to communicate effectively as part of a team in the salon as well as when carrying out a consultation with your client. Communication is an art that can be learnt and improved upon. Do it well and you will gain the trust and confidence of your client, ensuring a long-lasting professional relationship. Do it badly and you will probably never see your client again.

In the art of consultation and communication we will consider:

- **how to gain trust**
- **verbal and non-verbal communication**
- **physical communication**
- **understanding how people communicate differently**
- **communication with different client groups**
- **consulting with your clients**
- **identifying your client's needs and wishes**
- **using open and closed questions**
- **using visual aids**
- **advice and after-care**
- **pre-cutting hair tests**
- **skin, hair and scalp conditions**
- **facial shapes and features**

This chapter links to the following S/NVQ units

G7 Advise and consult with clients

G9 Provide hairdressing consultation services

INTRODUCTION

Consultation and communication with your clients are critical to ensure that you develop a relationship where you understand and trust each other. You need to understand all the different forms of communication – verbal, non-verbal and physical communication – to create an atmosphere where you and your client can openly discuss your client's requirements and expectations. You will need to take into account the client's face shape and features and the condition of their hair and scalp to ensure that the end result is always what your client is expecting and enhances their appearance and your professional image.

HOW TO GAIN TRUST

The *Oxford English Dictionary* defines the word trust as: 'A firm belief in the reliability or truth or strength of a person, a confident expectation.'

The salon you work in will have a visual and atmospheric impression to which your client has been drawn. It is up to you and the rest of the salon team to ensure that whoever enters the salon experiences what that impression portrays. The receptionist is often the first person the client encounters and it is important that they create the right impression for you to then build on.

When a client comes to the salon they are putting their trust in you as a professional stylist to carry out a service that meets their expectations. They are putting their trust in you. To keep that trust you must make sure that you build a rapport with your client. *Rapport* is defined as a sympathetic relationship or understanding between two people. Rapport cannot be touched or measured, but you know when it is there. Building rapport with your client starts the minute that you meet. How you communicate will determine how your client will perceive you. You can make a client feel special and comfortable during their visit or you can make them feel unwanted, uncomfortable and angry. You determine how your client will react by how you communicate through speaking, listening and using body language.

VERBAL, NON-VERBAL AND PHYSICAL COMMUNICATION

There are several ways to communicate with your clients: verbal communication (using your voice) or non-verbal communication (how you express information through body language). In addition to these types of communication, there is a third method that is used in hairdressing – physical communication. To communicate effectively you will need to use all forms effectively to ensure that you give the correct information to your clients.

Verbal communication

One-to-one verbal communication is an important skill that all hairdressers need. Your voice can expose your attitude and your emotions. A client will quickly identify your interest in them by the way you speak through the tone of your voice. To communicate effectively you should:

- speak clearly and unambiguously
- vary your voice tone and inflections
- speak with courtesy and confidence
- use professional vocabulary and not slang
- never speak while you are eating.

Non-verbal communication

There are many forms of non-verbal communication, the majority of which you will use in your everyday tasks as a hairdresser. These may include such things as:

- making an appointment or writing down a message
- gestures and facial expressions
- eye contact
- clothes and accessories.

When you are visually communicating with your client your message is delivered in three ways:

- body language
- tone of voice
- words.

Your body language will account for approximately 50 per cent of the information your client will receive. Your tone of voice will be approximately 40 per cent of the information you receive and the words you use will make up the remaining 10 per cent.

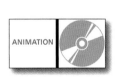

ANIMATION

How you communicate with your client

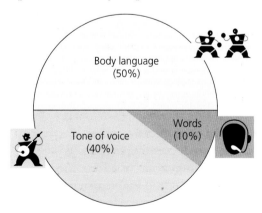

How you communicate with your client

As you can see from the pie chart, body language is a very important part of communication. The way you stand, make eye contact and use facial expressions will all give a message to your client about you, your attitude and your emotions, for example:

- a genuine smile lights up your face and conveys happiness and interest;
- eye contact lets clients know you are listening and interested in them;
- your head tilted to one side will indicate that you are interested.

Whereas:

- standing with hands on your hips can give the interpretation of aggression;
- crossing your arms can make you appear defensive.

Usually, if a client's body frame is loose or more widely spread they are generally relaxed or at ease. However, if your client holds their body in a stiffer or more together position they are usually experiencing nervousness, tension or discomfort, for example:

- a client touching their face is usually indicating anxiety;
- a client clenching their fist is indicating tension or aggression.

Being able to interpret these signals and act on them to reassure or relax your client will help to create a good relationship.

Clothing, jewellery and accessories are also forms of non-verbal communication. Each time you meet a new client you will make judgements about the way they look. The moment you look at your client, you take in information about their appearance, the clothes, the type of jewellery and accessories they are wearing. Some clients will have bold and vibrant accessories, which may give you an indication that they are adventurous and outgoing, willing to try new haircuts and styles. However, other clients may wear discreet, understated accessories and jewellery, which may give the impression that they would prefer a more classic look. This information is then used as part of your overall analysis during the consultation, to help build a picture of the types of styles that will suit and work well for your client.

Physical communication

This type of communication is different and restricted to those who provide a service that requires them to have physical contact with their clients. As a stylist, physical communication is an important part of building up trust with your clients. Clients know by the way you touch them if you are confident or unsure about what you are doing. A young hairdresser is often intimidated at the thought of physical contact with the client. They may express this at the shampooing stage by the way they wash the client's hair. They may fail to ensure the client's head is positioned correctly or may not use the correct amount of pressure when massaging the scalp. A positive touch will give the client confidence and tell them that you know what you are doing. A negative touch will give the impression that you are not sure of your own ability.

ACTIVITY

Practise different methods of communication with a colleague. Decide on a topic that you want to discuss and role-play it. During the role-play, take turns in using different methods of communication. Can you identify when your partner is using positive and negative communication?

Hairdressing is a profession which requires you to work within a client's personal space.

Putting your hand on your client's shoulder or arm during a consultation will help break down barriers. This will help the client feel more relaxed so that you can then carry out investigations of the hair and scalp prior to carrying out the cutting service. It is important that you physically check the hair and scalp for:

- hair growth patterns
- bumps or scars

that may affect the finished haircut. Identifying any problems at the consultation will enable you to discuss any alterations to the haircut.

UNDERSTANDING HOW PEOPLE COMMUNICATE DIFFERENTLY

Not everyone communicates in the same way. Some people are more expressive or flamboyant with their body language and expressions. Others may have a loud voice that booms or vibrates across a room. These characteristics could give you the impression that they are confident people. However, this is not always the case. Sometimes first impressions can be deceiving and it is not until you have had the opportunity to talk with someone and review other forms of communication signals that you can truly make a judgement.

It is part of your role as a good stylist to identify the best way to communicate with your clients to build a good relationship. For some clients this will be using visual aids such as style books to draw out information to help explain what they want. For others it will be listening carefully while they give you detailed information about themselves and what style they want.

COMMUNICATION WITH DIFFERENT CLIENT GROUPS

The way you communicate with your clients will often be determined by their age, disability, gender and culture.

If your client is a child don't forget to treat them as an individual during the consultation. You will be gathering information not only from their parent or guardian but also from the child. It is important to make them feel comfortable and encourage two-way communication. It is important to make eye contact and if possible talk to them at the same height level, which can be less threatening. Putting them at ease is important to encourage them to talk or respond to your questions.

Some clients may have a disability that you need to take into consideration to ensure that you are communicating effectively:

For people who are deaf or have a hearing impairment make sure you:

- have the person's attention before talking;
- look at the person you are talking to;
- don't mumble or eat while talking;
- use simple language and short sentences;
- turn down music or try to avoid background noise;
- use style books, visual clues and gestures;
- write down questions or responses if necessary.

For people with mobility limitations make sure you:

- sit at the same level
- make eye contact
- treat a wheelchair as the client's personal space
- talk naturally to the person in the wheelchair, not their companion.

For people with sight impairments make sure you:

- touch them on the arm to indicate you are there and going to talk to them;
- offer your arm to lead them to your styling station and the backwash area;
- make sure the area is free of any obstacles which they may trip over;
- make sure you use simple terminology that the client will understand when giving advice. Your client may not be able to see hand gestures and style images to help you explain the haircut;
- listen carefully to your client and ask questions to make sure you understand exactly what your client wants;
- if possible use touch to confirm the amount of hair to be cut off at the fringe or the overall length at the back.

Being aware of different cultures and not assuming that everyone is 'just like me' will give you a greater understanding of people and communication skills. Culture can refer to religion, social, political and family customs. To build a client relationship it is necessary to respect differences, do not make judgements but learn about different cultures so that you do not offend clients without realising it.

> **TIP** ✓
>
> Avoid conversations and stating an opinion on topics that are sensitive and could cause offence, such as religion, racial remarks, sex and politics.

Remember, everyone communicates differently. Some people will talk in short sentences that are structured and to the point, while other people like to tell a story that combines a lot of information. In this case you will need to listen carefully and extract the important facts needed to determine the haircut your client actually wants.

IT'S A FACT! !

Did you know that a gesture may have different meanings in different cultures?

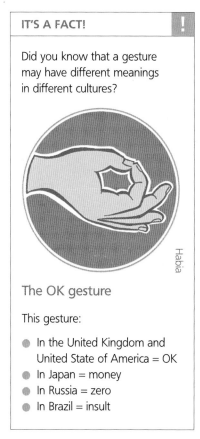

Habia

The OK gesture

This gesture:

- In the United Kingdom and United State of America = OK
- In Japan = money
- In Russia = zero
- In Brazil = insult

CONSULTING WITH YOUR CLIENTS

The aim of consulting with your client is to find out what your client's wishes are and if they can be achieved. To do this you need to:

- examine the client's hair and scalp;
- decide on the most suitable cutting techniques to use to create the desired result;
- decide on the most suitable cutting tools to use to achieve the desired result;
- decide what products will be needed and advise the client;
- advise the client on the maintenance requirements.

The consultation process is an important part of any service; get it wrong and you will have a dissatisfied and unhappy client. It is essential that you build a relationship with your client from the very beginning. Make sure you introduce yourself and show that you are curious about the client and their personal needs.

Your communication and listening skills need to be effective to ensure that you gather all the information you need to create an end result that meets your client's expectations.

Part of the consultation will take the form of an analysis of the hair and scalp. *Analysis* is the term used when you examine the hair and scalp to identify any disease or disorders that may affect the cutting service or a particular haircut. For example, if a client has a very strong hair growth pattern you may make recommendations for adapting or altering the hairstyle so that it will work better for the client.

Using open and closed questions

We all communicate with each other. The art is to communicate well so that we all understand each other. As described above there are many forms of communication that can be used to put a client at ease as well as to gather information. During the consultation it is important that all forms of communication are used, first to make the client feel welcome and relaxed – especially if they are a new client. This can be done by:

- smiling and introducing yourself;
- putting your hand on their shoulder or arm to help break down personal space;
- asking your client questions about their hair and lifestyle so that you can start to build up a picture of the type of hairstyles your client would prefer;
- using appropriate visual aids, such as style books;
- listening to your client's response.

During the consultation it is important that you ask a variety of different questions to ensure you gather the correct information. Some clients will find it easy to respond to your questions and will give you clear guidance on their hair and what they want doing, while other clients will find it difficult to explain and may feel a little intimidated by the salon environment. The use of open questions will help your client to explain any difficulties they may have with their current hairstyle and what changes they want.

Open questions

Open questions can start with any one of the following words:

- Who?
- What?
- Where?
- Would?
- When?
- How?

Any question starting with these words will automatically encourage your client to give you more information that a 'yes' or 'no' response. You will probably need to probe further with additional open questions to build up a full picture of your client's requirements, but by asking open and probing questions you will ensure that your client has given you the information needed to create a hairstyle that meets their wishes.

Examples of the types of open questions you can ask your client:

- How would you like your hair today?
- When did you last have your hair cut?
- Would you like to change your current hairstyle?
- Would you like me to make some suggestions?
- Would you like to look at a style book to help explain what your likes or dislikes are?
- Have you had any problems with your hair since your last visit?
- How much length do you want to keep?
- How long do you like your fringe?

Closed questions

Closed questions are used to gain a limited amount of response such as 'yes' or 'no'. They are useful to confirm your understanding of an earlier question or confirming the service with your client by repeating what has been agreed.

Types of closed questions you can ask your client:

- You are having a haircut today?
- Do you usually have your parting on the left?
- Do you want me to cut your hair around the ear?
- Do you want your hair any shorter?

When you have asked your client questions and listened to the response make sure that you confirm the information that you have heard to make sure that both you and your client have understood each other and are clear about the hairstyle agreed before starting the haircut.

Using visual aids

Using visuals aid during consultation can be another way of communicating with your client. Not all clients find it easy to explain how they would like you to cut their hair. Although you will ask open and closed questions to gather information, the client may find still find it difficult to express their thoughts, particularly if they are a new client to the salon and feeling a little intimidated.

Style books are a useful to help gather information. Use the style book to confirm your ideas such as:

- Do you want your hair to be as short as this at the sides?
- In this picture the style shows the hair a little longer at the sides – which do you prefer?

However, when using visual aids to confirm your client's requirements, make sure your client is agreeing to the aspects of the haircut within the picture and not the total image portrayed. For example, you may be showing your client the effect of a fringe within a hairstyle but your client is seeing a stunning-looking model and has not fully focused just on the fringe detail: their mind may be agreeing to the total image portrayed and not their individual requirements.

Advice and after-care

As part of your consultation with your client, don't forget to advise them on how to maintain their new style at home to achieve a similar look to the one you have created. Advice is not just about the styling techniques that you will use, which brush to use or how to use the straightening irons, it is about explaining how often the hair will need to be cut to maintain the style, whether other services such as colour will give the hairstyle more definition and which products you are using to create the look.

When talking about hair-care and styling products explain the features and benefits of the product to your client and let your client hold and smell the product. Explain to them how much to use and how to apply it to their hair. Tell them how long the product will last and how much it costs. Make sure you answer their questions honestly and do not claim that the product will do something that it is not supposed to do. The Trade Description Act 1972 states that products should not be falsely or misleadingly described in relation to its quality, price, fitness or purpose by advertisements, displays, orally or through descriptions. Your client will appreciate you giving them advice; it is then up to them to decide whether or not to take your advice on this occasion.

TIP

Make sure you listen to your client during the consultation and confirm information with them to show that you have understood. Remember that one of the main complaints from clients is that their stylist cut their hair too short and did not listen.

TIP

Take time when necessary during the haircut to explain what you are about to do, especially if you are working on the back sections of the hair.

IT'S A FACT!

A *feature* of a product is what it contains and how it works.

A *benefit* of a product is what it will do for the client's hair.

ACTIVITY

Take time to learn about the different styling and finishing products you have in the salon. With the help of a colleague practise your technique for giving advice and explaining the features and benefits of products to your clients.

PRE-CUTTING HAIR TESTS

Before you can begin your haircut you need to understand the characteristics of the hair you will be cutting. This can be done through the consultation and analysis stage where two important tests should be carried out: porosity and elasticity tests.

Porosity testing

This test is used to determine the condition of the hair. The cuticle, which is the outside protective layer of the hair, is made up of between four and eleven layers of overlapping scales. When hair is in good condition, the scales will lie flat and evenly down the length of the hair shaft, making the hair feel smooth and reflect light, and giving a glossy appearance. However, if the hair is in poor condition, the cuticle scales will be missing or damaged and will make the hair feel rough and look dull. Glossy hair is very important for some haircuts. For example, a classic one-length bob looks best if the hair is straight and glossy.

A porosity test is carried out on the hair before it is shampooed. You need to take a small bundle of hairs, holding the ends of the bundle together with one hand. Using the thumb and forefinger of the other hand you gently stoke the hair from the ends to the roots to feel the condition of the cuticle. If the hair feels smooth it means that the cuticle is laying flat and that the hair is in good condition. However, if the hair feels rough, it is an indication that the cuticle has been damaged and that the hair is in poor condition.

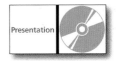

Porosity testing

IT'S A FACT!

The keratin structure of hair that is very curly, i.e. African-type hair, can also feel rough when a porosity test is carried out and may not give a true indication of the condition of the cuticle.

Elasticity test

When the structure of the cortex is in good condition it allows the hair to stretch under tension and, when the tension is removed, to return to its normal length and position. However, if the cortex has been damaged, the properties of elasticity will be reduced, or in extreme cases, completely missing. Recognising the amount of elasticity in the hair will be one of the determining factors for the decision of how much length should be removed during the haircut and whether to cut the hair wet or dry.

You must remember that hair will stretch more when it is wet than when it is dry. Therefore, if you are cutting hair wet you have to allow for the fact that once the hair is dry the length will appear shorter. This is particularly important when you are cutting hair at the fringe area or if the hair has curl or wave movement. For this reason it is often better to finish cutting the fringe after the hair has been dried, and you should be aware that curly and wavy hair will look shorter when the hair is dried.

To carry out an elasticity test take a single strand of hair and, supporting it at the roots to ensure the client's comfort, gently stretch the hair, then release it, observing how soon it returns to its natural position. Hair that is in good condition will stretch and then immediately return to its normal position. If the hair has reduced elasticity, the hair may return to its natural position

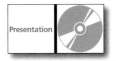

Elasticity test

more slowly. However, hair that is in very poor condition may stretch and not return or may break under the slightest pressure.

ACTIVITY

Carry out a range of porosity tests on a variety of different hair conditions and types. For example, compare the amount of elasticity there is in very curly hair to that of very straight hair. Also, compare how much the elasticity is reduced in hair that has chemical treatments with virgin hair. Then compare the porosity levels on a whole length of hair from the roots to the ends. You may find the condition of the cuticle at the roots is in good condition, but that the condition of the cuticle at the ends of the hair is poor.

SKIN, HAIR AND SCALP CONDITIONS

There are several hair, skin and scalp conditions that you need to be aware of prior to cutting hair. The most common are:

- infectious or contagious parasitic conditions
- hair defects
- scalp defects.

Infectious or contagious parasitic conditions

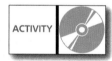

ACTIVITY

Hair, skin and scalp conditions

During the consultation it is important to identify any conditions of the hair, skin or scalp that may contra-indicate the haircutting process.

Such conditions could be caused by bacteria, fungus or a virus, or may be a parasitic condition. Such conditions can be transferred by direct or indirect contact.

Bacterial conditions

Condition	Cause and symptoms	Treatment
Impetigo Dr M. H. Beck	Bacteria enters an opening of the epidermis causing a burning sensation, which is followed by yellow or clear filled spots or pustules, which dry into yellow or honey-coloured crusty formations. The condition can be seen on any area of the body, but commonly on the face and scalp. Impetigo can be spread by direct or indirect contact by a person or through dirty tools and towels.	Medical treatment should be sought and hairdressing services should not be carried out.
Folliculitis Mediscan	Bacteria enters the opening of the follicle causing an infection. The opening of the follicle can be inflamed and painful. The condition can be seen on any part of the body or on the scalp. Folliculitis can be spread by direct or indirect contact with a person or through dirty tools and towels, or it can be caused by irritation from chemicals.	Medical treatment should be sought and hairdressing services should not be carried out.

Fungal conditions

Condition	Cause and symptoms	Treatment
Ringworm of the scalp Dr John Gray	The condition is not caused by a worm, as the name suggests, but a fungus that lives on the keratin of the hair and skin. The condition is also known as Tinea capitis. The symptoms are patches of pink skin surrounded by a red active ring. The centre of the patch is covered by grey scales of dead keratin and the stubble of broken hair.	Medical treatment should be sought and hairdressing services should not be carried out.

Viral conditions

Condition	Cause and symptoms	Treatment
Warts Mediscan	These outgrowths of the lower epidermis are caused by a virus and can be found anywhere on the body. They appear as small roughened areas of skin that grow into irregular-shaped lumps. They can vary in colour from pale to flesh-coloured to brown. The virus is more easily spread through water, so shampooing a client with warts on their head may lead to the transfer of the virus.	Medical treatment should be sought and hairdressing services should not be carried out.

Parasitic conditions

Condition	Cause and symptoms	Treatment
Head lice John Burbage/Science Photo Library BLM Health A nit (the egg of a louse)	This condition is also known as Pediculosis capitis. Small insects, which are parasites, head lice live by sucking and feeding on the blood of their host. The lice live on the scalp and lay eggs called nits. The nits are glued onto the hair shaft with a special cement near the roots of the hair, or in areas where the hair is abundant, for example within the bands holding pony tails or under hair bands – anywhere the eggs will be least noticed and most protected. The nits are clear in appearance while the louse forms inside, but turn white and are easily visible once the louse has hatched and the egg shells have dried. Head lice are caught through head-to-head contact.	Pharmacist treatment should be sought and hairdressing services should not be carried out.
Scabies Dr M. H. Beck	This condition is caused by the itch mite. The mite, called Sarcoptes scabiei, burrows through the skin leaving greyish lines and reddish spots. The condition is extremely itchy particularly at night. Scabies is contagious and can be passed on by close physical contact.	Medical treatment should be sought and hairdressing services should not be carried out.

Hair defects

Condition	Cause and symptoms	Treatment
Fragilitis crinium Dr John Gray	This condition is the splitting of the hair shaft at the ends of the hair – split ends. It is caused by chemical, physical or environmental damage to the hair and can be prevented by regular cutting and conditioning treatments.	Cutting to remove the split and damaged ends of hair and using conditioning treatments to prevent future damage. Advise the client how to physically treat their hair during drying and styling.
Trichorrhexis nodosa Dr John Gray	This condition is similar to fragilitis crinium, but the splitting occurs along the hair shaft, rather than the ends of the hair. It is caused by chemical, physical or environmental damage to the hair and can be prevented by regular cutting and conditioning treatments.	No treatment can cure this condition, but the client should be advised to have conditioning treatments to prevent future occurrences. Advise the client how to physically treat their hair during drying and styling.
Monilethrix Redken	This condition is often referred to as *beaded hair*, this is because the hair has bead-like swellings and constrictions along its shaft. The hair can be very weak and often breaks close to the scalp. The condition is caused by irregular development of the hair within the hair follicle.	No treatment can cure this condition, but the client should be advised to have conditioning treatments that may help protect the hair. Advise the client how to physically treat their hair during drying and styling.
Damaged hair Dr John Gray	Hair can be damaged at the cuticle and/or the cortex. Some damage will manifest itself as fragilitis crinium or trichorrhexis nodosa, but other times the symptoms can be dull, rough, porous or dry hair.	Deep reconstructive conditioning treatments can aid this condition, and the client should be advised to have regular, follow-up conditioning treatments to prevent future occurrences. Advise the client how to physically treat their hair during drying and styling.

Scalp and skin defects

Condition	Cause and symptoms	Treatment
Sebaceous cysts Mediscan	These are non-infectious lumps that appear on the scalp. The lumps are caused by a blockage of the sebaceous gland leading to excess sebum filling up under the surface of the skin.	Medical advice should be sought, but hairdressing services can continue.
Pityriasis capitis Dr P. Marazzi/Science Photo Library	This condition, commonly known as dandruff, is excess shedding of the epidermis, which leads to small flakes of loose dry skin on the scalp that can drop and become visible on the shoulders. The dry scales are not infectious and can be caused by irritation to some hairdressing products or a excessively dry scalp. However, if the scales become oily and sticky it is a sign that a fungal infection is present.	Providing a fungal infection is not present, dandruff can be treated by using medicated shampoos and moisturising the scalp. Hairdressing services can continue.
Psoriasis Mediscan	This is a non-infectious condition which can be distressing for the client. The real cause is unknown, but is thought to be related to stress and the overproduction of epidermal cells. The symptoms can be seen as raised red patches covered in white or silvery scales.	Some specialised shampoos can help or the client may be referred to a trichologist.
Seborrhoea	This non-infectious condition of the skin and hair is caused by the overproduction of sebum which makes the hair very greasy and lank. This condition can make the hair very difficult to work with as physical work such as blow-drying or chemical services can stimulate the production of sebum.	Regular washing with a specialised shampoo can help or the client may be referred to a trichologist.
Keloids Dr John Gray	This non-infectious condition of the skin is most commonly found in clients who are African Caribbean. Keloids are small raised scars that can often be itchy. They can be caused by cutting the hair too close to the skin either when cutting around the hairline or when shaving.	Moisturise the skin regularly.
Alopecia Dr Andrew Wright Alopecia areata	The generic term for hair loss is *alopecia*, but there are different types that can affect the hair on the scalp and the body. The cause of some types of alopecia are unknown, though can be linked to stress-related illnesses and changes in hormone levels. Alopecia areata appears as small round or oval patches of hair loss, which can spread to total loss of hair on the scalp – alopecia totalis – if the condition worsens and the bald patches join together. Traction alopecia is caused by excessive tension on the hair, leading to hair being pulled from the scalp leaving areas of baldness. This is commonly seen following braiding of the hair or incorrectly applied hair extensions – especially around the front hairline. Cicatricial alopecia is caused by damage to the dermis following physical injury or damage. The hair follicle is damaged and scarring prevents the growth of new hair.	Clients with alopecia should be referred to a trichologist for specialised advice. Traction alopecia can be prevented by reducing the stress on the client's hair and providing advice about how long braids or hair extensions should be worn for.

FACIAL SHAPES

Each and every client will have a unique and different facial shape and bone structure. You must be able to identify the shape of your client's face during the consultation stage in order to make recommendations about the shape of the haircut. The finished style must complement the shape of the client's face and their facial features.

The most common facial shapes are:

- oval
- round
- square
- rectangular
- long
- heart or triangular
- pear
- diamond.

Each of the facial shapes will have defining characteristics that help you to identify what your client has.

Oval	
Habia 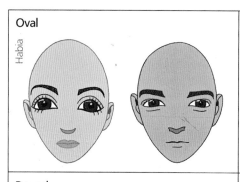	An oval face is described as the perfect shaped face. The face is evenly balanced with the overall appearance likened to the shape of an egg. The forehead will be slightly wider than the chin. The length of the face will be slightly longer than the width. The jawline will be slightly curved, but not angular. Any hairstyle suits this shape of face.
Round	
Habia 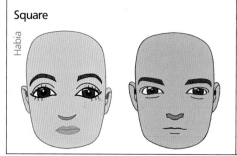	The proportions of a round face are equal in length and width and the jawline will be rounded. Hairstyles that create length and reduce the width of the face are best for this facial shape.
Square	
Habia	The proportions of a square face are equal in length and width and the jawline will be angular in shape. Hairstyles that create length to the face and soften the angles of the jawline are best for this facial shape.

Rectangular Habia 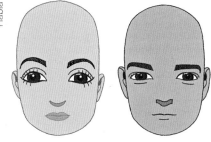	The jawline of a rectangular face will be angular and the length of the face will be longer than the width of the face. Hairstyles that soften the angular jawline and reduce the length of the face are best for this facial shape.	
Long Habia 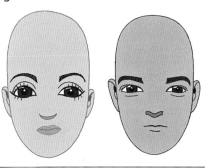	The length of a long face will be longer than the width, but the jawline will be curved and not angular. Hairstyles that reduce the length of the face are best for this facial shape.	
Heart or triangular Habia 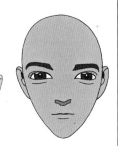	A heart-shaped or triangular face will be wider at the forehead and curve into a narrow chin. The face will be equal or slightly longer in length than it is in width. Hairstyles that reduce the width of the forehead and create the illusion of width at the chin are best for this facial shape.	
Pear Habia 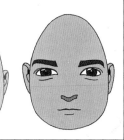	A pear-shaped face is the exact opposite of a heart- or triangular-shaped face. In this case, the forehead will be narrow, but the jawline, which can be angular or curved, will be wider. Hairstyles that reduce the width of the jawline and create the illusion of width at the forehead are best for this facial shape.	
Diamond Habia 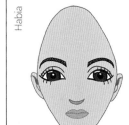	The forehead and chin will be narrow, but there will be width at the cheekbone area creating a diamond-shaped face. Hairstyles that create width at the forehead and jawline will be best for this shaped face.	

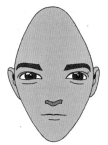

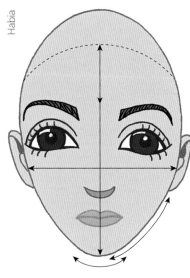

Identifying the shape of the client's face

Identifying the shape of the client's face

To correctly identify the shape of your client's face you need to look at the:

● length of the face from the top of the forehead to the chin;

● width across the face from ear to ear;

● shape of the jawline – is it angular or curved?

● height and shape of the forehead;

● shape of the chin.

The length and width of the face will give you an indication of the overall shape. If the face is slightly longer than it is wide it is likely to be oval. However, if the width and length are equal in length it is likely to be round or square. A face that is much longer than it is wide is likely to be long or rectangular.

The shape of the forehead and jawline also influences the identification of the facial shape. An angular jawline will be linked to a square, rectangular or pear-shaped face, whereas a curved jawline will be related to a round, oval, long or pear-shaped face.

A pointed chin can indicate a triangular or heart-shaped face.

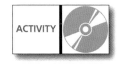

Identify the shape of the client's face

ACTIVITY	
Work with a colleague and identify the shape of each other's faces.	

Changing the appearance of the facial shape

The most perfect facial shape is considered to be oval. This means that you can create any haircut and finished style the client with the oval facial shape chooses. However, with careful cutting and styling, the illusion of an oval face can be created. Therefore, if the client asks for a hairstyle that is not suitable for their facial shape, you need to be able to either adapt the style they have chosen, or provide suitable alternatives. Do not be afraid to tell your client that the style they have chosen is not suitable – though be careful about the way you tell them. Your client will be pleased that you have taken the time and trouble to give them a haircut and finished style that is exactly right for them.

Creating length to the face

Making the face look longer is matter of optical illusion. A centre parting can create the illusion of length as can height at the top of the finished hairstyle. Heavy fringes should be avoided, but soft, fine textured fringes can be used as you will still be able to see the forehead, preventing the face from being further shortened.

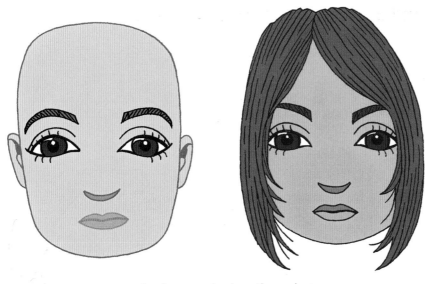

How the appearance of a face can be lengthened Habia

Reducing the length of the face

Partings that run diagonally to the forehead or are off-centre can reduce the length of the face. Keeping the hair flat at the crown area will also reduce the length of the face. Fringes are a great way of disguising a high forehead.

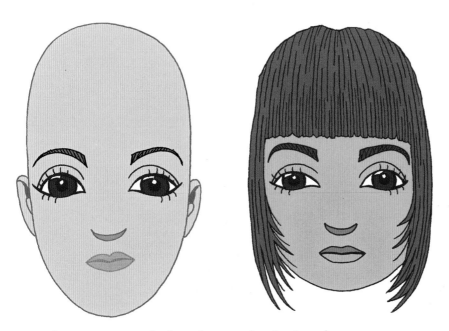

How the appearance of a long face can be shortened Habia

Creating width to the face

Cutting the hair shorter or styling the hair away from the face at the sides will increase the width of the face.

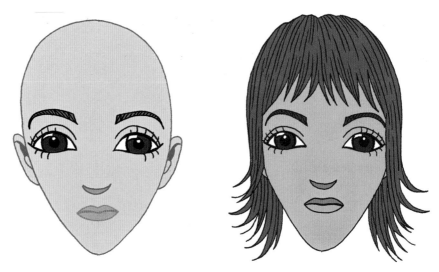

How the appearance of a narrow face can be made wider Habia

Reducing the width of the face

Cutting the hair so that it is texturised to lie on the sides of the face will reduce width.

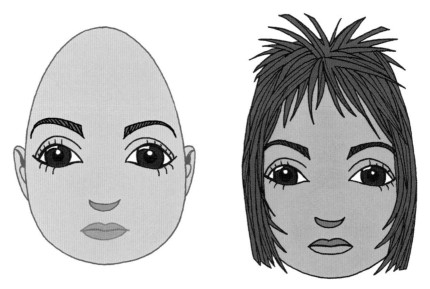

How the appearance of a wide face can be made narrower Habia

Head shape

Once you have decided on your client's face shape it is important that you determine your client's head shape. Not all clients have the same shape of head. Some clients will have prominent occipital bones or bumps on the head. Other clients will have a flat crown or a flat occipital area. You will need to take these features into consideration before starting your cut. If your client's head is flat you will need to consider the angle at which you should cut the hair and, if additional hair length is required, the angle that will give the head more shape, particularly if you are going to create a short hairstyle.

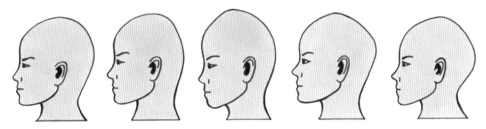

Head shapes Habia

Assessment of knowledge and understanding

Test yourself on the content of this chapter by answering these questions.

Assessment activity level A

Complete the table and state if the hair and scalp conditions listed are infectious or non-infectious.

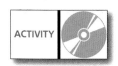

Identifying infectious and non-infectious hair and scalp conditions

Condition	Infectious, or non-infectious
Fragilitis crinium	
Psoriasis	
Sebaceous cyst	
Alopecia areata	
Head lice	
Impetigo	
Warts	
Tinea capitis	
Folliculitis	
Trichorrhexis nodosa	
Seborrhoea	
Monilethrix	
Scabies	
Keloids	
Damaged hair	
Pityriasis capitis	

The answers to this activity can be found at the end of the book.

Assessment activity level B

Look at the following illustrations of different facial shapes and identify the shape.

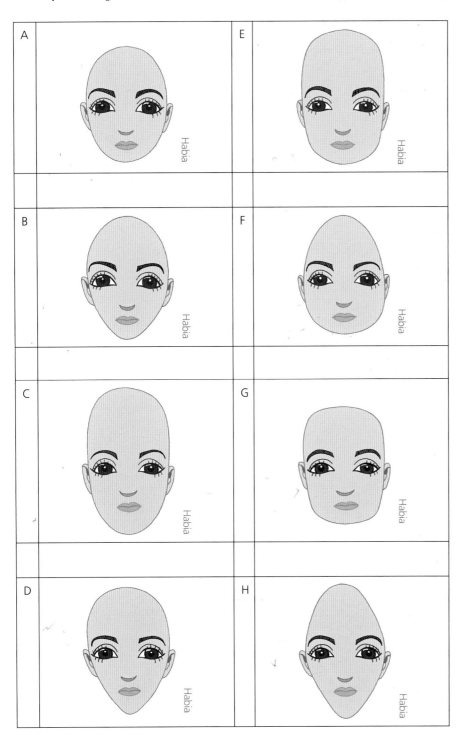

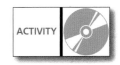

ACTIVITY

Identify the different facial shapes

The answers to this activity can be found at the end of the book.

Assessment activity level B

1 What is meant by the term *trust*?

2 What is meant by *effective communication*?

3 Give three examples of verbal communication.

4 Give three examples of non-verbal communication.

5 When communicating with your client name the three ways in which your message is delivered to your client.

6 List the percentage for each of the three methods your message will be received by the client.

7 What is *consultation*?

8 What does the term *analysis* mean?

9 List three topics of conversation with your clients that should be avoided.

10 Explain the difference between open and closed questions.

The answers to this activity can be found at the end of the book.

Assessment activity level C

Produce a style book that can be used as a visual aid for clients that is categorised into hairstyles and haircut shapes for the different facial shapes.

Assessment activity level C

Design a leaflet that can be given to clients who during the consultation have been found to have head lice.

The leaflet should be sympathetic in nature, provide advice about the removal of lice and nits, and stress that they are welcome back in the salon as soon as they have cleared the infestation.

Assessment activity level B

Complete the table below. In the first column list eight essential attributes for effective communication. In the second column give an example of how you have used them in your work.

Effective communication	Example of effective communication

The answers to this activity can be found at the end of the book.

Assessment activity level C

Neurolinguistic programming (NLP) examines different ways people think, feel and communicate with one another, and how this can build relationships.

Research and write a report on how NLP works and how it can be used in the salon to build relationships with other team members and your clients.

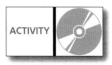

ACTIVITY

Crossword

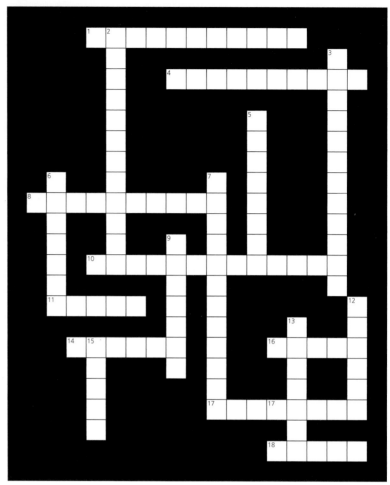

Across

1. Accept
4. Impression based on understanding
8. Head to head?
10. Judgement of a situation
11. A belief in a person
14. Method used to gain information
16. Sounds forming elements of speech
17. Making contact
18. Expression of non-verbal communication

Down

2. Used to gather information prior to starting service
3. The way you stand
5. Query
6. Harmonious communication
7. Another term for partnership
9. Opposite of speaking
12. See communication
13. Make sure the information is correct
15. A representation of the salon environment

The answers to this activity can be found at the end of the book.

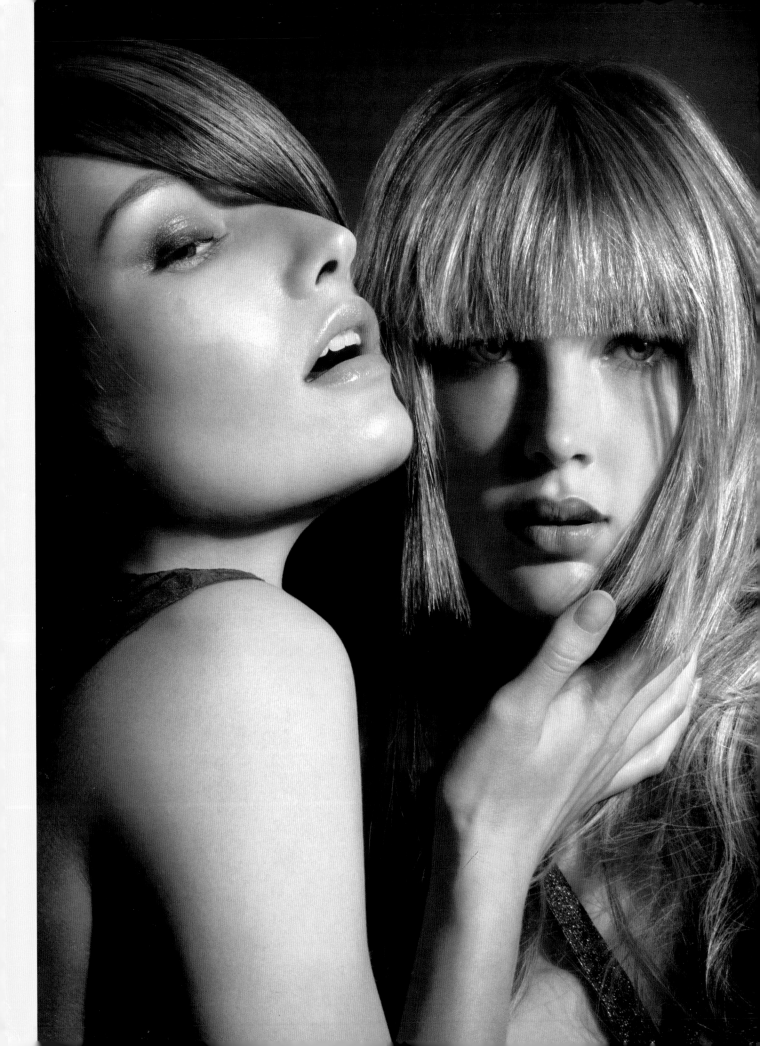

tools, equipment
and products

Your tools will become a part of you. I've had my primary pair of scissors for over twenty years and they are an integral part of my technique.

MARK HILL

chapter 4

TOOLS, EQUIPMENT AND PRODUCTS

Learning objectives

In this chapter, you will learn about the different types of tools, equipment and products available for cutting and shaping hair. Understanding about the variation in tools and equipment for cutting, and when and how to use them, will help you to achieve the results your clients expect from you. Ever heard the saying 'a bad workman always blames his tools'? Well, if you understand how to choose and use the right tools to achieve the result your client is after and look after them correctly this will never apply to you. Today more than ever products are a vital 'tool' when cutting. Products can help control and manipulate hair to make it easier to handle when cutting or will create definition, shine and texture to bring the hairstyle to life once it has been dried. In tools, equipment and products we will consider:

- **types of tools and equipment used for cutting hair**
- **how and when to use the different types of tools and equipment**
- **how to handle cutting tools**
- **cleaning and maintaining tools and equipment**
- **health and safety requirements**
- **new developments in cutting tools**
- **products used during cutting and styling**

This chapter links to the following S/NVQ units

H6 Cut hair using basic techniques

H7 Cut hair using basic barbering techniques

H21 Create a variety of looks using barbering techniques

H22 Design and create patterns in hair

H27 Create a variety of looks using a combination of cutting techniques

INTRODUCTION

Have you ever tried to cut something without using a pair of scissors? You can try cutting with a knife but if the blade is not very sharp it is difficult and very rarely successful. Hairdressing is about being artistic, but without the right tools you will never achieve complete success. You ask any celebrity hairdresser and they will tell you that they cannot achieve a good result without using the correct tools and products. Having the correct scissors is a personal thing; choosing a pair of scissors that suit you in size and balance is the key to a happy haircutting relationship.

TOOLS AND EQUIPMENT USED FOR CUTTING HAIR

Scissors

Scissors are your most important purchase as a hairdresser. It is important that you choose the right scissors for you.

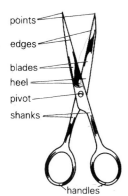

points
edges
blades
heel
pivot
shanks
handles

Parts of a pair of scissors

When choosing scissors it is important to ask yourself a number of questions before buying them:

- What type of scissors do I need?
- What size scissors do I need to buy?
- What type of scissor blade do I need to buy?
- What type of shank and handle do I need?
- Which cutting techniques will I be able to use with the scissors I buy?
- How should I look after my scissors?

Types of scissors

There are different types of scissors available on the market; they all vary in size, style and cost. It is up to you to decide on the best pair for you, the type you need and how much you are going to spend. When you first start cutting hair you may not want to buy top-of-the-range scissors until you have practised your technique and got use to handling scissors correctly.

Serrated scissors The fine serrations on the edge of the blades will stop the hair from sliding down the blade. This is useful to help control the hair when you first start cutting but will usually pull on the hair if you try to slide the scissor blades down the hair shaft when using some texturising cutting techniques.

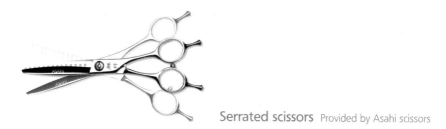

Serrated scissors Provided by Asahi scissors

Straight scissors Convex blades are the sharpest for slicing and chipping in to the hair. The better the quality of scissor the easier it is for the blades to slide and cut through the hair.

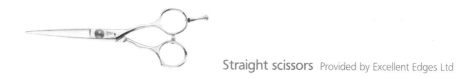

Straight scissors Provided by Excellent Edges Ltd

Texturising scissors These scissors can be used to thin out the hair and also add texture and definition to the hair design during cutting. There are a variety of texturising scissors available that have different spaces between their teeth so they will remove varying percentages of hair. Practice and experience will be needed to ensure you do not remove too much hair at any one time to spoil the overall design of the haircut.

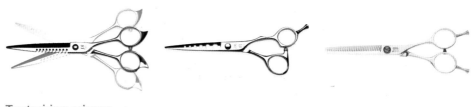

Texturising scissors

Provided by Asahi scissors   Provided by Excellent Edges Ltd   Provided by Asahi scissors

Thinning scissors Thinning scissors are used to remove bulk from the hair, while leaving the original length.

IT'S A FACT! !

Thinning scissors are also known as *aesculaps scissors*.

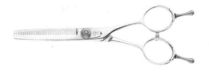

Thinning scissors Provided by Excellent Edges Ltd

There are two types of thinning scissors:

- one blade notched
- both blades notched (these will remove less hair than a scissor with the one blade notch).

Although thinning scissors are a good choice to start with when you first start cutting, and will remove bulk and weight from the hair, you need to use them carefully and thoughtfully if you want to produce a great hair design.

What size of scissors do I need to buy?

One way to measure a pair of scissors to make sure they are right for you is to measure the scissors from the tip of the blade to the end of the longest handle. The scissor should lie in the palm of your hand with the finger hole of the longest handle touching the base of your thumb and the tip of the scissor blade resting in the last section of your middle finger. However, always make sure that you hold the scissors and play with them to make sure that they feel balanced and comfortable in your hand before buying them.

Whatever the size of the scissors you choose you need to make sure that they feel comfortable in your hand and are easy to control. Some stylists will prefer to have a variety of different-sized scissors available so that they can alternate their scissor choice depending on the haircut they will be carrying out.

What type of scissor blade should I buy?

Most types of European scissors are designed with a bevelled edge, which means a flat section is machined on to the scissors, which are often serrated. Bevelled-edged scissors are made from a mixture of metals which makes them light to use. Convex-bladed scissors are the sharpest blades, similar to the blade of a razor. They are mainly made from steel such as stainless steel. However, some companies will have specialist steel developed for them to use; an example being Jaguar who use micro-carbide steel, which stays sharper and is extremely wear-resistant. The higher the quality of steel the more expensive the scissors are to buy, but if looked after and serviced properly they will last you a lifetime. The more expensive scissors will usually have additives put in to the steel such as cobalt and molybdenum to give the blades added strength, or high-carbon steel which has a high resistance to corrosion and wear. The pivot or screw system at the centre of the scissor holds the blades in place and controls the tension on the scissors. The tension can be adjusted by altering the pivot or screw system.

The cost of the scissors will depend on the quality of the steel and the type of screw system used. The more expensive the scissor the more sophisticated the screw system may be; for example, it may set, control and stabilise the tension of the scissors.

Habia

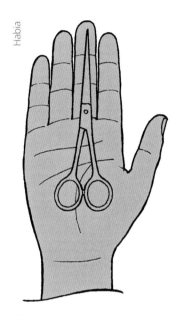

Finding the correct size of scissor to use

IT'S A FACT! !

To check the correct tension for scissors you need to let the blades open and then allow one blade to freely drop to become closed. If the blade stops before closing leaving the blade at about ten to the hour position the tension is correct.

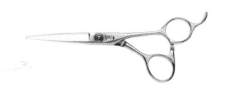

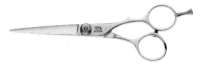

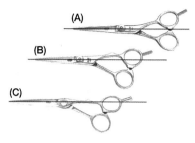

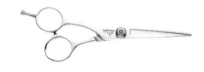

Provided by Excellent Edges Ltd

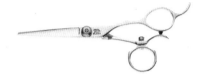

Provided by Excellent Edges Ltd

Kasho scissors – handle configuration

Provided by Excellent Edges Ltd

Provided by Excellent Edges Ltd

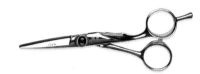

Provided by Asahi scissors

Scissors with different types of handles and shanks

What type of shank and handle do I need?

There are scissors available with either right- or left-handed handles. When you start cutting it is important that you choose to use the most comfortable type of handle for you; for example, if you are left handed it will be more comfortable to use left-handed scissors. If you learn to cut hair using right-handled scissors it can be difficult and uncomfortable to change to left-handled scissors.

There are three main shank and handle designs available:

- The *even handle*, the handles of which are symmetrical.
- The *offset handle*, one handle of which is longer than the other. This allows the stylist's arm and elbow to be in a lower position during cutting which makes it more comfortable and helps prevent repetitive strain injury.
- The *crane*. This is the most modern design. It is similar to the offset handle but this design relieves stress on both the stylist's shoulder and wrist.

Razors or hair shapers

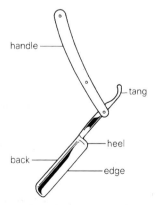

Parts of a razor

Razors or hair shapers are used to:

- remove weight by tapering the ends of the hair
- create texture and definition to a haircut
- clean away hair from the neckline or hairline to give clean lines.

Razors are also used in barbering for shaving.

Disposable blades

A razor with a disposable blade is often referred to as a *hair shaper*.

Disposable bladed razors or hair shapers are the hairdresser's most popular choice of razor for cutting hair because they are light to hold and easy to maintain since a new blade is used for each new haircut. The old blade is disposed of in a sharps box to meet health and safety regulations.

Solid blade

A solid-blade razor is also known as a *fixed blade*. This type of blade must be sharpened regularly by a method called honing and stropping. Solid blade razors are not often used because they are difficult to sterilise and many local health and safety authorities do not allow their use.

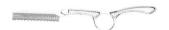
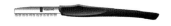

Feather razor Provided by Excellent Edges Ltd

Designing razor Provided by Kasho

Guards

Razors and hair shapers often have a removable guard that protects the cutting edge of the blade. This guard can be used to determine the amount of hair to be removed when cutting the hair or be used to protect the blade when not in use.

> **TIP**
>
> Never cut dry hair with a razor. It will pull on the hair shaft and be uncomfortable for your client.

Clippers

Electric clippers and trimmers

Electric clippers and trimmers are powered either directly from mains electricity or by using electricity to recharge battery-operated clippers. They are quick to use and are more accurate than hand-held clippers (see below). They are used to create outline shapes and definition in a haircut and are often used in barbering for short haircuts using the technique clipper over

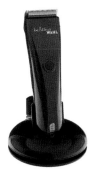
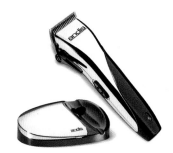
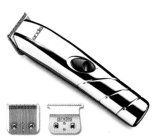
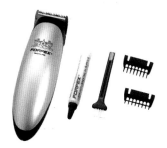

Wahl electric trimmer
Image courtesy of Wahl (UK) Ltd

Andis electric trimmer
Image courtesy of Andis

BaByliss electric trimmer
Image courtesy of BaByliss

comb. The Wahl Super Taper is one of Wahl's bestsellers; its ergonomic design and durability makes it ideal for continual everyday use. Clippers are now available in different sizes so that you can choose the best size for a particular haircut. For example, small narrow clippers or trimmers are often easier to use when removing hair from the neckline or for creating intricate patterns or lines in the hair. The BaByliss Palm Pro Tramliner, for example, is designed to be battery powered and fit snugly into the palm of your hand to give you freedom to create precise, tailored lines in the haircut. The Andis T Liner II Combo Rechargeable Cordless Trimmer/Clipper is also battery operated and designed to fit comfortably in the hand giving good flexibility during cutting. It comes with a T-blade for precise trimming and clipper blades and attachments for styling and general clipper cutting.

Clippers may have different speed settings, enabling you to control the motor speed for different hair types. For example, the BaByliss Forfex Cord/Cordless Clippers are a multi-purpose clipper with two speed settings. Normal speed allows for ultra smooth cutting on fine hair while the high speed increases the cutting power for coarse, thick hair. The Andis Shaper Clipper is cord/cordless and rechargeable; it has a powerful rotary motor and is contoured to fit comfortably into the hand. The Wahl Bellissima is a mains-rechargeable clipper that contains an intelligent microchip controlled rotary motor that gives constant cutting power, adjusting to the thickness of the hair. The Wahl Bella rechargeable trimmer is slimline and lightweight and very quiet with snap on/off blades for easy cleaning and blade maintenance.

Clippers have different blade sizes and types that are used for different haircuts.

- The number 000 is used to remove all unwanted hair; for example, when creating hairline shapes.
- The detachable texturising and razor blade is used for creating texture in a haircut.
- The 'T' blade used for intricate outline work such as creating patterns in the hair.

The BaByliss Forfex range has a clipper that has a snap-in blade with a ceramic cutter that stays cooler and sharper than conventional steel blades.

Clippers often come with a variety of different sized detachable clipper comb attachments.

Clipper comb attachments

Detachable clipper comb attachments enable the hair to be cut to a predetermined length. They enable you to work quickly and accurately. The attachments come in a variety of sizes:

- Number 1 attachment – leaves the hair 3 mm long.
- Number 2 attachment – leaves the hair 6 mm long.
- Number 3 attachment – leaves the hair 9 mm long.
- Number 4 attachment – leaves the hair 12 mm long.

- Number 5 attachment – leaves the hair 16 mm long.
- Number 6 attachment – leaves the hair 19 mm long.
- Number 7 attachment – leaves the hair 22 mm long.
- Number 8 attachment – leaves the hair 25 mm long.
- Number 10 attachment – leaves the hair 32 mm long.
- Number 12 attachment – leaves the hair 38 mm long.

Number 2 and 3 tend to be the most popular comb attachments used, particularly in barbering.

Hand clippers

This type of clipper cuts the hair in the same way as the electric clipper, however they are not often used in the salon today as the electric clipper is quicker and the variety of sizes and safety features make electric clippers easier to use. Hand clippers are operated by squeezing the handles together which in turn moves the upper blade to cut the hair.

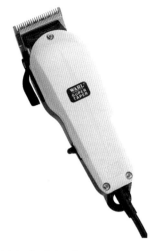

Wahl electric clipper
Image courtesy of Wahl (UK) Ltd

Image courtesy of Wahl (UK) Ltd

TIP

Clipper blade attachments may vary between different manufacturers so check the manufacturer's guide before cutting the hair.

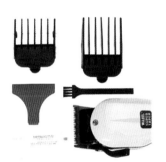

Detachable clipper comb attachments

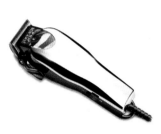

Andis electric clipper
Image courtesy of Andis

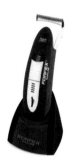

BaByliss electric clipper
Image courtesy of BaByliss

Combs

Cutting comb

Cutting combs are usually straight combs that have two different sizes of teeth, one fine and the other coarse. The fine teeth are used to give control when cutting and allowing the hair to be closely cut to the scalp.

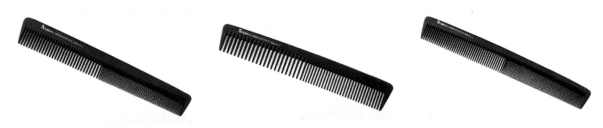

Cutting combs Denman

The coarser or wider teeth are used for combing the hair into position. The cutting comb varies in flexibility. For example, when using the scissor-over-comb cutting technique the comb needs to be flexible and thin so that it bends to the shape of the head; while, when cutting long straight hair, the teeth can be wider and less flexible. If you are cutting very curly or African-type hair you may need to use a wide-tooth cutting comb or afro comb so that you do not damage the hair and can comb the hair into shape easily when cutting the hair in to a style using a freehand cutting technique.

HOW TO HANDLE CUTTING TOOLS

Holding scissors

The correct way to hold your scissors is with the thumb in one handle and the third finger in the other handle. This gives you more control of the scissors as you work. During cutting, when the scissors are not in use you should remove your thumb from the scissor handle and cradle the scissors in the palm of your hand. The third finger still holds the scissors in place with the blades closed but enables you to work with the comb in the same hand while you hold your scissors. When using your scissors make sure that the handle of the scissor is not pushed to far down your thumb as this will restrict your movement when cutting. Only the thumb moves during the cutting process allowing that blade to move against the second blade which remains still at all times.

Habia

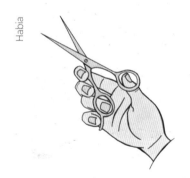

How to hold your scissors

ACTIVITY	
Practise handling your scissors: open and close the blade by only moving your thumb.	

ACTIVITY	
Practise removing and replacing your thumb from the scissor handle and holding your cutting comb in the same hand.	

TIP	
Visit a hairdressing trade show such as Salon International so that you can try out different types and styles of scissors before you buy.	

Holding a razor

You need to be careful when opening your razor or hair shaper as the blade is very sharp. Keep one hand on the base of the razor handle and the other one on the back shoulder so that your fingers are away from the blade. Hold the razor with the thumb on the underside of the shank away from the heel and the little finger resting on the tang. The remaining fingers should rest along the top of the back shank to give you balance and allow you to safely move the razor in different directions.

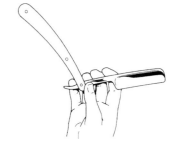

How to hold your razor

TIP	
Always keep the razor closed to cover the blade when the razor is not in use.	

TIP	
When passing the razor make sure that the razor is closed, wrap your hand around the razor to prevent it from opening and pass the razor with the tang facing away from you but towards the person you are passing it to.	

Holding clippers

Electric clippers vary in weight and size. It is important that you use clippers that are secure and comfortable for you to hold and balance easily in your hand whilst working. Rechargeable clippers tend to be lighter and small to hold and are more versatile to use as they do not have a wire attached.

Holding a cutting comb

When you hold your cutting comb for the majority of cutting techniques make sure that you are supporting each end and that the comb is balanced. When using the scissor-over-comb technique the comb is held at one end between the index finger and thumb so that you can direct the comb and tilt the angle as you work up the head.

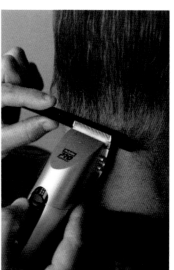

Habia

How to hold a clipper

CLEANING AND MAINTAINING TOOLS AND EQUIPMENT

How do I look after my scissors?

Caring for your scissors is important to ensure that you do not damage or blunt them. After each use you need to:

- Wash and dry your scissors or wipe the blades with a spirit to remove hair clippings, and then sterilise them.
- Try never to drop them as this can offset the balance of the scissor or damage the blades.
- Never use your scissors for anything other than cutting hair as this will blunt the blades more quickly.
- Avoid lending your scissors to others as this will offset the balance.
- Oil your scissors regularly using proper scissor oil.
- Always store your scissors in a protective pouch.

Scissors need to be serviced at least once a year, but many professionals will ensure their scissors are in perfect condition by having them serviced every three months. Your scissors are your main asset to achieving a perfect haircut; therefore, do not let just anyone service them. Make sure they are serviced by a professional hairdressing scissor sharpener. These companies can often be found at hairdressing trade shows. Alternatively, you can send your scissors back to the manufacturer. If your scissors are not sharp they will damage the hair.

How do I look after my razor?

- Try never to drop your razor as this will damage the cutting blade.
- Clean and sterilise it after use.
- To prevent corrosion of any metal parts remove moisture and oil regularly with fine oil.
- Always store your razor in a protective pouch.

How do I look after my electric clippers?

- Try never to drop your clippers as this will offset the balance and damage the cutting blade.
- Clean and sterilise the blades after use.
- Always check that the top blade is not protruding over the lower blade as this could cut the client's skin.
- To prevent corrosion of any metal parts remove moisture and oil regularly use fine oil.
- Make sure that the plug is secure before use.

- Store the clippers in a safe place when they are not in use.
- Use a protective guard over the blades when they are not in use.

How do I dispose of sharps?

All used blades should be kept away from general salon waste and disposed of separately by placing them in a safe secure-topped container. When the container is full it can be disposed of. Your local authority may provide a collection arrangement for your sharps box. You should contact your local council offices for advice.

Methods of sterilising tools and equipment

Sterilisation is the complete eradication of living organisms. Tools and equipment must be cleaned and sterilised before using them on your clients. As part of the consultation you will be identifying the tools and equipment you will need for the haircut. This will be combs, scissors, possibly a razor or clippers, and it is up to you to ensure that they are ready to use and fit for purpose.

There are three main methods of sterilising or disinfecting tools. They are:

- heat
- radiation
- chemicals.

Within the hairdressing salon this will equate to:

- heat = the use of an autoclave
- radiation = the use of an ultraviolet light box
- chemicals = the use of barbicide.

Heat

Autoclaves are the most reliable method of sterilising but are not often used within the salon. They work by building up steam pressure creating heat that destroys all living bacteria. They are used for sterilising tools such as your scissors. If you want to sterilise your combs by this method they must be able to withstand the very high temperature produced by the autoclave.

Radiation

The ultraviolet (UV) light box is often used as a method of sterilising cutting tools. You must wash and dry the tools before placing them in the box. The ultraviolet light will prevent bacteria growth on the tools but complete sterilisation is not guaranteed as tools will only be sterilised on the areas that the UV rays reach: the tools must be turned over to ensure they have been exposed to the light on all sides. Because this method of sterilising is time-consuming and sterilisation cannot be guaranteed it is often better to use the UV light box as a hygienic method of storing tools that have already been sterilised by another method, rather than storing them in your tool bag.

Chemicals

Using chemicals is the most common method in the salon of disinfecting cutting tools. In hairdressing a chemical known as *barbicide* is frequently used. It is a clear, blue, low-level disinfectant. It does not sterilise tools but reduces the probability of infection. Barbicide must be changed daily and all the tools must be totally submerged in the solution and left in the solution for the time recommended by the manufacturer.

Different tools and equipment are cleaned disinfected and sterilised in different ways.

Most suitable method of cleaning, disinfecting and sterilising tools and equipment	Scissors	Razors	Electrical Clippers	Clipper blades	Combs and attachments
Wash thoroughly with hot soapy water and then dry	✓	✓	✗	✓	✓
Use of autoclave	✓	✓	✗	✓	✗
Use of ultraviolet radiation	✓	✓	✗	✓	✓
Use of chemicals/disinfectants such as barbicide	✓	✓	✗	✓	✓

Health and safety

It is important that you know how to use your tools and equipment safely so that you do not injure yourself or your clients and colleagues. Making sure that you know what you are doing, are trained to use your tools and equipment safely and correctly and know how to look after and maintain the tools and equipment is the responsibility of both you and your employer. You must make sure that you only use clean, sterilised tools and equipment on your clients, that the equipment is in good working order before you use it and that you report any faults such as loose wires on electric tools to the designated person in the salon. The equipment should then be removed from the salon floor and labelled as faulty and stored safely until repaired by a qualified professional electrician. There are a number of health and safety regulations in place to protect you and your clients; for example the Provision and Use of Work Equipment at Work Regulations (PUWER) (1998) are for employers and requires that equipment such as electric clippers provided and used at work in the salon be:

- suitable for its intended use
- safe to use, maintained and if required inspected to ensure it is safe for use
- only used by staff that have received adequate information, instruction and training.

For further information see Chapter 7.

NEW DEVELOPMENTS IN CUTTING TOOLS

Glass hair designer

The FB1 glass hair designer designed by Frank Bisson is a new cutting tool that is suitable for cutting any style on all types of hair.

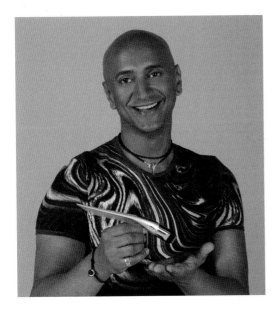

The FB1 glass hair designer with inventor Frank Bisson Frank Bisson

Its features include:

- designed for both left- and right-handed hairdressers;
- a tail for sectioning;
- a curved comb that fits every angle and curvature of the head. This comb is heat resistant and can be used with straightening irons. The spacing of the comb teeth allows the comb to be used on African, European, Oriental and Asian type hair;
- a glass blade for cutting the hair;
- a protective cap for the glass blade for protection when carrying it around;
- an ergonomic design that makes it comfortable to hold.

The glass blade is extremely sharp and has a serrated end with many cutting angles. The cutting edges are within these serrations, which makes it safe to touch the blade. However, for health and safety reasons avoid contact with the cutting edge of the glass blade. The hair that slides between the serrations will be cut.

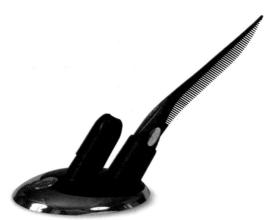

The FB1 glass hair designer
Frank Bisson

The sharpness of the blade means that no damage is caused to the hair, eliminating split ends. It gives each strand of hair a tapered end to help increase the softness and blending of hair throughout the haircut, which is ideal for:

- blending layers and additional hair such as extensions;
- giving volume and body to fine hair;
- producing a soft geometric line;
- creating textured, scrunch-styled and spiky haircuts;
- dealing with awkward growth patterns and controlling unmanageable hair;
- twisting and cutting hair to give extra volume, body and texture and to achieve creative effects such as giving straight hair a wavier appearance;
- cutting hair close to the scalp;
- cutting at awkward angles around the scalp.

Like the blade of a razor the glass blade of the FB1 glass hair designer should be replaced after each client to maintain hygiene.

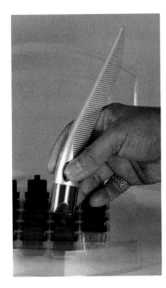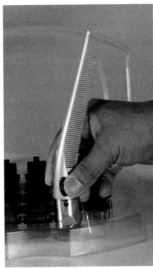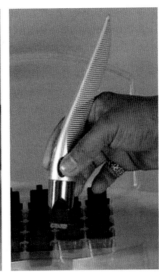

Glass blade Frank Bisson

How to use the FB1 glass hair designer

The FB1 should be held like a pen. If you are right handed, you should hold it so that the comb teeth point towards your left-hand side. If you are left handed, you should hold it so that the comb teeth point towards your right-hand side. By holding it in this way the comb section can be easily used by turning your wrist.

When using the FB1 designer the side of the glass with the cutting edge should be nearest the hair. For best results the hair should be cut wet and only used on dry hair for finishing touches to the haircut. There are three main glass cutting techniques:

- **Cross-cutting** – Gently press the cutting edge against the section. At the same time apply a slight lateral motion in order to cut across the section. This technique can be used with the cutting edge at different angles to the hair. The cutting angle can be varied so that you can achieve either blunt or graduated sections. For added texture you can cross-cut through the section with a slight chopping motion. A geometric line can be achieved by cross-cutting a series of small sections.

- **Sliding** – Press the cutting edge against the hair and slide down along the section of hair. This technique is used for graduating a section of hair from short to long. The cutting angle can be varied to achieve different levels of graduation. You can apply this sliding technique with a chopping motion in order to give a more shattered and textured effect along the section of hair.

- **Scraping** – Gently scrape the cutting edge along the section. This technique is used for thinning and weight removal. At the same time it will give lots of texture. The amount of weight removed can be varied in two ways. First, by changing the angle of the cutting edge (a steeper angle will give less thinning), second, by applying different amounts of pressure (more pressure will result in more thinning).

The techniques can be used by cutting the hair in a downward motion by holding the hair section down or you can cut the hair in an upwards motion with the section of hair held up.

To hold the hair sections, a section of hair should be held between the tips of your index finger and thumb with tension applied. You can also hold the section of hair between your fingers in the conventional way. The techniques can be used on straight or twisted sections of hair to achieve different effects.

TIP
When using the FB1 glass designer it is extremely important that you apply tension to the hair whilst cutting.

Ultrasonic hot razor

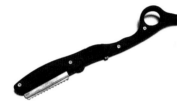

The Ultrasonic Hot Razor is a new design of razor that uses heat. Although using a razor can produce great effects in a hair cut, the razor can often cause damage to the hair, especially when used over a long period of time. The Ultrasonic Hot Razor helps to eliminate split ends caused by a razor. It produces ultrasonic vibrations which, combined with the heated blade, allow a clean cut on both wet and dry hair while sealing the cuticle. The Ultrasonic Hot Razor has three cutting options:

- heated vibrating blade
- vibrate only
- regular cut.

This helps increase your control and precision and is particularly good for cutting hair extensions.

Courtesy of American Dream

The Ultrasonic Hot Razor

Thermo Cut System

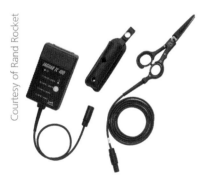

Courtesy of Rand Rocket

Thermo Cut System

The Thermo Cut System is a range of cutting tools that include scissors, thinning scissors and razor. They have constantly heated blades which automatically seal the ends of the hair during cutting. This helps to retain the natural moisture in the hair and protect against environmental influences. Used regularly the system will help reduce split ends, creating manageable hair. The range of tools allows you to apply all the cutting techniques to create different cutting effects. The system has adjustable temperatures to suit different hair types and conditions.

TIP
Make sure you have enough spare tools to work on other clients while you are sterilising tools used on a previous client.

The SAFE-System

The SAFE-System is a patented scissor system invented by Cyril Gallie of Scissor Safe Ltd and produced by Tondeo. The SAFE scissor has a shortened and rounded tip on one of the blades. The design of the blades helps to reduce the risk of any cutting injuries to yourself or to your client, especially when using point-cutting or contour-cutting techniques. The scissors have low soft-polished blades with a wide blade angle and are good for creative slicing techniques as well as being stable and giving a good grip. The blades are available in two blade sizes of 5.0 or 5.5. Although the blades are different lengths this will not interfere with your cutting technique or your cutting performance and can be used by both beginners and experienced stylists.

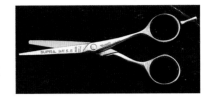

The SAFE-System

PRODUCTS USED DURING CUTTING AND STYLING

Technology in hair products has advanced quickly in the last 25 years. Today, there are a wide variety of products available to protect, strengthen, reduce or maximise curl, add moisture to dry hair or even to create shine on dull dry hair. No matter what condition your client's hair is in, there will be a product available to help achieve the result you are after. Products can be used to aid cutting and help make hair more pliable and easy to manage; examples are leave-in conditioners and styling lotions that add moisture and increase the natural strength of the hair.

Understanding the different types of styling products used in your salon will help you to select the right one for a client's hair type and the styling result you are after. To ensure your client can then re-create the style at home you need to explain why you have chosen to use particular products. Explain how and when to use the product, how much to use and the features and benefits that it has to offer. You can explain why your salon uses a particular range of professional styling products and that the salon retails them for the client to purchase and use at home. Clients often want to touch and smell a product so either give them the product to hold and smell or apply some on their hands so that they can experience the product for themselves. Your clients will be pleased that you have taken time to explain and recommend products for use: after all, a hairdresser's recommendation is the number one reason a client purchases a product. Clients may not always buy the product when you show it to them but you have given them a professional consultation that will encourage them to return to the salon for further appointments and to buy products.

TIP
Always keep yourself up to date with your product knowledge. Read the manufacturer's instructions on how and when to use a styling product to achieve the best results.

TIP
Don't just sell to your client but use your knowledge of the salon's product range to advise and recommend a product to meet your client's needs.

ACTIVITY

Review the styling and finishing product range in your salon. Identify the products that are best used to achieve:

- soft, medium and strong styling support
- moisture retention
- additional strength to the hair
- added shine to the hair
- environmental protection e.g. from the sun or from swimming
- heat protection e.g. from styling equipment
- definition to finished styles.

Different types of styling and finishing products

The table below gives a guide to the different types of styling and finishing products available for professional use and what they are mainly used for. Many products can be used in combination with each other to help you provide the result you and your client want to achieve the total look.

Type	Soft support	Medium support	Strong support	Added volume	Protect	Smooth/ straighten
Styling spray			Laquetrix	tecni.art texture spray/tecni.art pli	tecni.art fix anti-frizz	

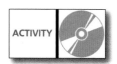

ACTIVITY

Match the styling and finishing products with their main use

Type	Soft support	Medium support	Strong support	Added volume	Protect	Smooth/ straighten
Protective spray		Redken Spray Starch 15			tecni.art hot style constructor	tecni.art hot style constructor
Moulding crème	tecni.art play ball pearl whip	Redken Roughpaste 12	tecni.art play ball beach crème			tecni.art liss control + /tecni.art colour show liss cream
Mousse		tecni.art volume lift	tecni.art full volume extra/tecni.art volume lift	tecni.art full volume extra/ tecni.art volume lift		
Gel		tecni.art play ball motion gelée/play ball pure jelly	tecni.art a.head glue	Biolage Gelée		

Type	Soft support	Medium support	Strong support	Added volume	Protect	Smooth/ straighten
Paste		tecni.art a.head web	tecni.art play ball density material/ tecni.art play ball deviation paste	tecni.art play ball density material	Redken Smooth Down Heat Glide	Redken Straight 05
Pomade	Redken Water Wax 03	tecni.art gloss wax				
Shine glaze	Redken Vinyl Glam 02	tecni.art hairmix glam definition	tecni.art glass control			
Polish	Redken Outshine 01					

Type	Soft support	Medium support	Strong support	Added volume	Protect	Smooth/ straighten
Shaping lotion	Redken Satinwear 02	Redken Thickening Lotion 06	tecni.art play ball extrême honey			
Hairspray		tecni.art fix move/ tecni.art color show finish spray	tecni.art air fix/ tecni.art fix design/ tecni.art fix anti-frizz			
Serum	série expert lumino contrast serum	tecni.art hairmix sublime shine				

Type	Soft support	Medium support	Strong support	Added volume	Protect	Smooth/ straighten
Shine spray	tecni.art crystal gloss	tecni.art gloss control				
Moulding mud			tecni.art a.head clay			
Cutting lotions	série expert hydra repair					
Wax	tecni.art color show define wax		fliktrix			

Type	Used during cutting	Used during styling	Used to finish
Styling spray		tecni.art pli	Biolage Finishing Spritz
Protective spray		tecni.art hot style constructor	Biolage Thermal-Active Setting Spray
Moulding crème	tecni.art liss control/ tecni.art colour show liss cream	tecni.art liss control + /tecni.art colour show liss cream/tecni.art hair mix supreme smooth	tecni.art play ball beach crème
Mousse	série expert volume extreme	tecni.art full volume extra/tecni.art volume lift/tecni.art color show volume mousse	
Gel		tecni.art play ball motion gelée	tecni.art play ball extrême honey/tecni.art play ball pure jelly/tecni.art a.head glue

Type	Used during cutting	Used during styling	Used to finish
Paste		tecni.art play ball deviation paste material/ tecni.art play ball density	tecni.art play ball deviation paste/tecni.art a.head web
Pomade		Redken Water Wax 03	tecni.art gloss wax
Shine glaze		tecni.art hairmix glam definition	tecni.art gloss control
Polish		Redken Outshine 01	tecni.art crystal gloss
Shaping lotion		tecni.art pli	ShapeTrix
Hairspray			AirTrix/tecni.art fix anti-frizz

Type	Used during cutting	Used during styling	Used to finish
Serum		tecni.art hairmix sublime shine	tecni.art liss control + /série expert extrême serum
Shine spray			color.smart reflective shine spray
Moulding mud		Redken Rough Paste 12	DirtyTrix/tecni.art a.head clay
Cutting lotions	série expert hydra repair		
Wax			tecni.art color show define wax

Assessment of knowledge and understanding

Test yourself on the content of this chapter by answering these questions.

Activity Level A

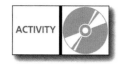

Answer the questions

1 Name the parts of a pair of scissors.
2 Which part of the scissors should stay still during cutting?
3 What is the purpose of the screw system?
4 Name the parts of a razor.
5 Name the three methods used for sterilising cutting tools.
6 Which is the best method of sterilising tools?
7 What is the purpose of comb attachments?
8 What type of scissor blade is best used for slide cutting?
9 Why would you use a razor during a haircut?
10 How do you safely pass a razor to someone?

The answers to this activity can be found at the end of the book.

Assessment activity level B

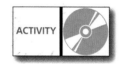

Fill in the missing word

Using the words listed below, answer the following questions.

1 The most important purchase a hairdresser buys is a pair of ___scissors___

2 Scissors with ___serrated___ blades will stop the hair from sliding down the blade.

3 Thinning scissors and ___texturising___ scissors both thin out and remove bulk from the hair.

4 _____ blades are the sharpest scissor blades.

5 The _____ is the part of the scissor that holds the blades in place.

6 Hair shapers are used to remove weight by _____ the ends of the hair.

7 The box used to dispose of blades is called a _____ box.

8 The three methods of sterilisation are heat, chemical and

_____.

9 Styling products can protect the hair from _____ damage.

10 A good hairdresser will always _____ to their client the correct styling product to use at home to maintain their hair between visits to the salon.

Convex	Pivot	Recommend	Serrated	Tapering
Environment	Radiation	Scissors	Sharps	Texturising

The answers to this activity can be found at the end of the book.

Assessment activity level C

Research and produce a report on the different types of cutting tools available on the market. Include in your report:

- the different types of scissors, clippers and razors available;
- the main features and benefits of the different types of scissors, clippers and razors available;
- what materials are used to manufacturer scissors;
- how the cost of scissors, clippers and razors compare across manufacturers;
- which scissors, clippers and razor you would choose to buy and why.

Assessment activity level A

Using the words listed below, label the two diagrams:

1 a pair of scissors

2 a razor.

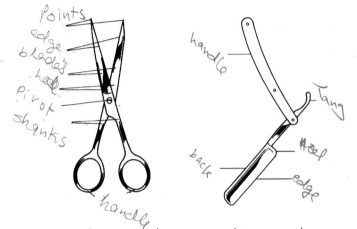

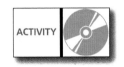

Label the diagrams of a pair of scissors and a razor

Back	Edge	Handle	Heel	Pivot	Shanks
Blades	Edge	Handle	Heel	Points	Tang

The answers to this activity can be found at the end of the book.

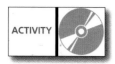

ACTIVITY

Word search

S	W	L	G	W	I	V	R	K	H	T	E	N	S	I	O	N	Q	K	V	S	C	W	N	D	P	J	I
T	L	T	B	Z	O	W	S	O	L	G	U	I	K	I	B	C	E	B	O	O	I	X	I	O	R	W	G
E	A	J	N	H	D	P	K	R	J	F	U	T	U	C	R	I	A	H	M	E	H	T	E	S	F	F	O
R	G	A	V	E	S	S	C	D	O	T	H	N	O	S	D	V	Z	B	O	A	U	E	M	S	H	L	C
I	Q	E	V	T	M	I	G	H	I	S	O	F	T	M	B	B	A	V	I	B	L	O	W	D	G	B	T
L	P	B	C	B	L	P	Z	I	Q	G	S	F	F	N	N	T	D	R	X	B	L	X	W	R	J	E	Q
I	J	C	S	U	L	R	I	W	B	L	D	I	J	N	T	T	S	W	A	S	W	W	Q	A	G	V	Q
S	P	P	C	N	T	Z	Y	U	B	V	E	Z	C	A	K	H	O	E	O	Y	P	Y	X	U	X	E	H
A	J	F	R	X	J	T	A	X	Q	K	K	C	C	S	A	Q	G	O	R	X	H	L	L	G	X	L	C
T	E	J	E	N	Y	S	I	J	S	E	P	H	V	P	G	R	K	F	L	B	A	O	P	C	N	L	I
I	S	B	W	Q	D	K	K	N	R	D	M	H	E	C	A	N	F	Y	L	S	N	K	T	Z	P	E	G
O	V	X	S	K	E	Y	O	Q	G	E	R	R	V	H	O	T	I	A	C	S	D	X	Y	O	L	D	X
N	N	E	Y	U	L	X	X	R	N	C	O	I	C	H	Q	R	K	N	A	C	L	I	E	O	E	E	B
I	Q	F	S	A	Y	N	B	T	O	B	O	E	A	X	V	P	R	R	N	Q	E	K	R	N	H	D	Z
L	C	A	T	S	O	I	S	D	J	Z	R	M	F	H	D	R	J	O	E	I	P	V	M	A	U	G	U
V	U	I	E	C	T	O	B	P	K	G	A	U	B	X	M	Y	G	O	S	B	H	R	H	E	X	E	J
C	D	S	M	I	H	B	H	L	X	F	G	R	C	D	M	T	X	T	S	I	R	T	F	Y	R	Z	H
S	V	R	J	S	A	T	P	R	U	N	C	E	Q	V	Y	C	K	R	X	U	O	A	S	V	M	M	T
H	S	I	R	S	V	U	E	P	Q	N	J	V	T	Q	N	V	L	L	C	K	J	N	B	H	K	L	O
O	E	A	Q	O	T	I	D	Z	Q	Y	T	A	F	F	Z	R	L	P	K	T	I	O	C	K	M	Z	P
T	L	B	P	R	Z	W	W	B	T	E	X	T	U	R	I	S	I	N	G	S	C	I	S	S	O	R	S
A	Y	D	R	S	U	Y	C	D	E	T	A	C	H	A	B	L	E	U	C	O	C	D	K	U	B	J	B
N	P	J	C	S	R	E	P	P	I	L	C	C	I	R	T	C	E	L	E	Z	W	B	V	X	K	G	D
G	M	L	X	B	Z	I	U	P	E	J	C	O	F	G	M	Z	I	Z	F	D	F	I	I	U	Y	E	M
M	V	X	C	W	F	H	C	U	O	P	E	V	I	T	C	E	T	O	R	P	B	U	B	J	D	S	J
B	N	W	G	V	N	Y	H	V	D	Z	U	X	Z	U	C	G	Y	Y	L	B	L	A	D	E	S	C	I
G	J	S	P	A	S	X	V	G	B	M	S	K	U	I	S	M	N	N	X	E	J	R	M	W	G	X	S
X	G	E	B	D	D	L	Z	R	N	A	Y	U	V	P	S	R	E	P	P	I	L	C	D	N	A	H	I

scissors	hairshaper	razor	blades
electricclippers	handle	haircut	sterilisation
cuttingcomb	texturisingscissors	equipment	tools
thinningscissors	handclippers	bevellededge	screwsystem
tension	barber	guards	combattachments
tang	blunt	offset	protectivepouch
corrosion	rechargeable	detachable	

The answers to this activity can be found at the end of the book.

Assessment activity level C: Crossword

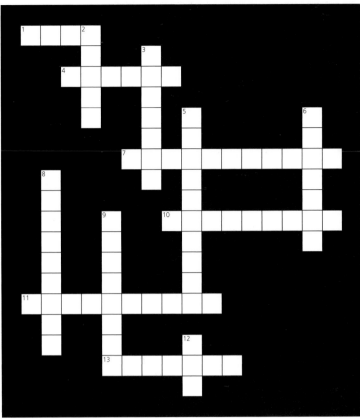

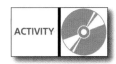

Crossword

Across
1. Part of a razor
4. Part of your scissors
7. Creates variation in length
10. Used to dispose of blades (two words)
11. Form of razor (two words)
13. Cutting method

Down
2. Protects
3. Rechargeable cutting tool
5. Type of blade
6. Required when cutting hair
8. Used for sterilising
9. Cutting tool
12. Lubrication

The answers to this activity can be found at the end of the book.

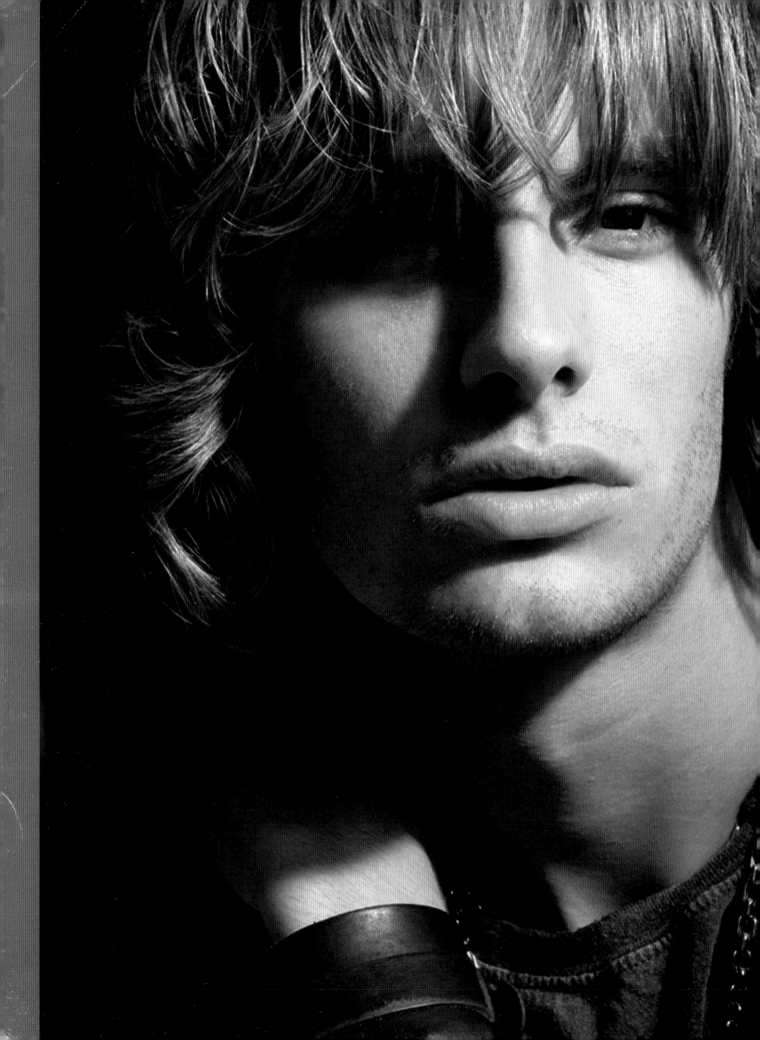

cutting techniques

> A successsful haircut depends on a good consultation, which should be 50 per cent about the hair and 50 per cent about what the client wants. It is important to ask your client the correct questions, the ones I ask are listed below. Then instil them with confidence. I never start a haircut until the client says: 'I trust you.'

ANTOINETTE BEENDERS, GLOBAL CREATIVE DIRECTOR OF AVEDA

Antoinette's client questions

1 How tall are you? What are your proportions?
2 What is your personal style?
3 How much time do you spend on your hair each day?
4 What do you like about your hair?
5 What do you not like about your hair?
6 What products do you use?
7 How often do you want to get your hair cut?
8 What is your lifestyle?
9 Does your hair need to be versatile?
10 Answer 'yes' or 'no' to these questions: Do you want your hair to be . . . Sporty? Trendy? Glamorous? Sexy? Fashionable? Elegant?

chapter 5

CUTTING TECHNIQUES

Learning objectives

In this chapter you will learn about the following:

- **cutting terminology**
- **the use of angles for haircutting**
- **cutting techniques and effects for hairdressing and barbering**
- **cutting looks**
- **neckline shapes**
- **how to cross check and balance a haircut**
- **how to individualise a haircut**
- **how styling, colouring and perming can be used to enhance or support a haircut**

This chapter links to the following S/NVQ units

H6   Cut hair using basic techniques

H7   Cut hair using basic barbering techniques

H21 Create a variety of looks using barbering techniques

H22 Design and create patterns in hair

H27 Create a variety of cutting looks using a combination of cutting techniques

INTRODUCTION

Actually carrying out a haircut on a real client for the first time will probably be the most exhilarating and yet most frightening experience that you ever go through in your hairdressing training. Unlike styling hair, once a hair has been cut, it cannot be replaced, and must grow back to its original length.

Therefore, every cut you make must be carefully calculated, planned and visualised before you begin in order to ensure that you achieve your client's wishes. By doing this you will go through three different stages.

- Stage 1 is to find out your client's requirements. You will do this through effective client communication and consultation. You can read about this in Chapter 3, The Art of Communication, where you will learn how to use verbal, non-verbal and other methods of communication. In this chapter you will also see that communication with your clients is a critical factor when cutting hair.

- Stage 2 is to identify the individual characteristics of your client's hair. If you do this, you will be able to confirm whether the client's requirements can be achieved. You will have read about analysing the characteristics of your client's hair in Chapter 2, Hair and Skin Structure and Analysis. In addition to analysing the type texture, density and length of hair, you need to take other factors about the client into consideration. For example, you need to be able to recognise the client's facial, head and body shape to ensure the haircut complements the individual features.

- It is only when you have these first two steps in place that you can begin Stage 3 – that of the actual haircut. For this stage you need to know how to choose the most appropriate cutting techniques and methods to achieve the desired outcomes of the haircut. You will read about these techniques in this chapter.

CUTTING TERMINOLOGY

When cutting hair, as with other aspects of hairdressing and barbering, there are certain words and phrases that you may never have used before. Therefore, before we look at the techniques for haircutting, here are some of the words and phrases that are included within this chapter and their definitions.

Hairdressing – this is the term that is used to describe the services that are carried out on hair, which includes haircutting.

Barbering – this is the term that is used to describe the services that are carried out exclusively on men's and boys' hair, which includes haircutting.

Basic cutting techniques – these are the techniques that you will develop when you first begin to cut hair, of which there are three for hairdressing. They are:

- club-cutting
- freehand cutting
- scissors over comb.

There are more basic cutting techniques for barbering. They are:

- club-cutting
- scissors over comb
- clippers over comb
- freehand
- thinning.

> **IT'S A FACT!** !
>
> Many of the cutting techniques that are carried out in hairdressing are also used in barbering.

Cutting techniques and effects – these are the techniques that you will use to create a variety of different effects once you have mastered the basic cutting techniques. For hairdressing they are:

- graduating
- layering
- tapering
- club-cutting
- scissors over comb
- clippers over comb
- thinning
- freehand
- texturising.

When barbering you will use the following techniques to create effects on the hair of men and boys:

- tapering
- club-cutting
- scissors over comb
- clippers over comb
- thinning
- using a razor
- freehand
- texturising.

Cutting looks – this means the overall finished hairstyle that is achieved from the haircut. The looks you will create when you first learn to cut are:

- one-length looks
- uniform layer
- graduation on long and short hair
- looks that include a fringe.

For barbering you will begin with:

- uniform layer
- graduation
- looks with and without a fringe
- looks with and without a parting
- looks that expose the ears.

When you have mastered the techniques to create the basic cutting looks, you will then be able to be more adventurous with your cutting techniques to create looks that fit into the following categories for hairdressing:

- classic
- current
- emerging.

And for barbering, you will create looks that fit into the following categories:

- traditional
- current
- emerging.

Cutting angles – to create the different haircuts you will hold and cut the hair in a variety of angles. The angles you use will range from 0° to 180°. A commonly used term in cutting terminology is a *right angle*, which means that the hair is held at an angle of 90° from the scalp.

Interior or exterior – this describes an area of the haircut on the head. The *interior* of a haircut refers to the hair that covers most of the head from the top, over the crown and down to below the occipital bone.

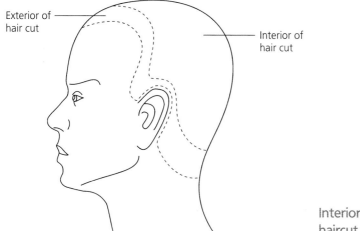

Exterior of hair cut

Interior of hair cut

Interior and exterior of haircut Habia

The *exterior* is the hair that follows the hairline that runs all around the head from the front hairline, over the ears and at the nape.

Critical influencing factors – these are the aspects that you must consider before you begin and during a haircut. The critical influencing factors will be different for each client, so every consultation must be individual. The critical influencing factors that must be considered for hairdressing and barbering are:

- hair density
- hair texture
- head and facial shape
- hair growth patterns
- hair elasticity
- hair length
- the client's requirements
- the client's lifestyle.

IT'S A FACT! !

When using barbering techniques you must ensure that you identify the same critical influencing factors as for hairdressing, but you also have to consider the effects of the presence of added hair and male pattern baldness on the final look of the haircut.

HOW CUTTING ANGLES AFFECT THE HAIRCUT

The *Oxford English Dictionary* describes an angle as 'a space between two meeting lines or surfaces'. In the case of haircutting, an angle is the space measured between the scalp and how far away from the scalp the hair is lifted before it is cut.

Angles are measured in degrees and are marked by a ° symbol. The number of degrees tells you how wide the space is. A full circle has 360°. In haircutting you will often hold the hair at angles of between 0° and 90°, but you will also use angles ranging from 90° to 180°.

To measure an angle you use a protractor, but this is not practical when you are cutting a client's hair. Therefore, you must be able to visually judge the angle of the hair as you lift it from the scalp. For example, a 90° or right angle looks like this when it is drawn on a flat surface:

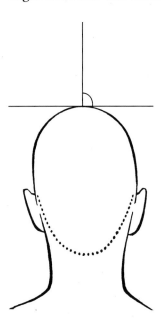

A right angle has 90° Habia

But, when you use the same angle on a head, which has a curved surface, you have to visualise it like this:

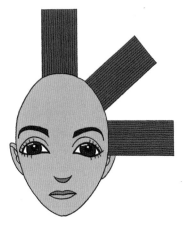

Hair held at 90° at the sides, top and back of the head Habia

Using angles in haircutting

Before you can begin a haircut, you have to be aware of how to hold the hair during the haircut. Hair is held a variety of angles, ranging from 0° to 180° depending on the look you wish to create, or the cutting technique you are using. When you are very experienced at cutting hair, you will be able to experiment and see that hair can be held at any angle, and each angle will produce a different effect. However, it is important, especially at the beginning, that you are able to recognise some of the most basic angles in which the hair should be held.

When to use a 90° or right angle

The right angle is one of the most commonly used angles when cutting hair, but the most crucial one when cutting a uniform layered look.

A *uniform layered haircut* is one that can be very short, short, medium or even very long. The significant aspect of the cut is that the layers are exactly the same length all over the head.

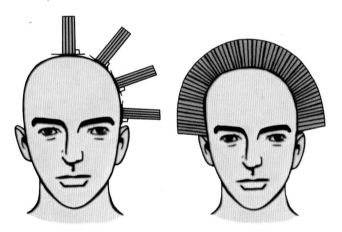

Uniform layer cutting projections Habia

To achieve this you must consistently hold the hair at a right angle and follow the natural shape and contours of your client's head. You can see 90° angles being used in Chapter 6 in the step by step: uniform layer.

When you hold the hair during a uniform layered haircut, you must change the position of your hands to ensure that you follow the shape of the head.

At the back of the head you hold the hair like this:

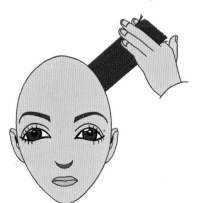

Holding hair at right angles at the back of the head Habia

> **TIP** ✓
>
> Right angles are mostly associated with squares, but of course your client's head is not square, but curved – so, when you are calculating how to measure a right angle on a curved surface, you have to imagine a straight line lying over the top of the curved surface.

On the top of the head you hold the hair like this:

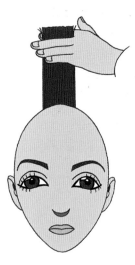

Holding hair at right angles to the top of the head Habia

At the side of the head you hold the hair like this:

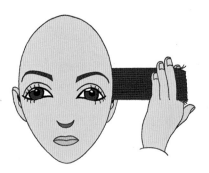

Holding hair at right angles to the side of the head Habia

When to use a 45° angle

Angles of 45° are commonly used during graduation. The term *graduation* refers to hair that has been cut so that it gives the effect of gradually changing in length from long to short and from short to long. This means that the length of the hair within the interior of the haircut will be longer or shorter than the lengths of the exterior.

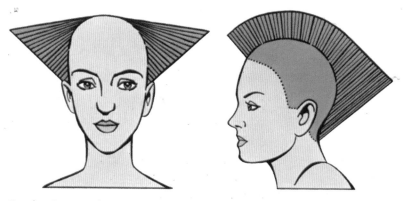

Graduation cutting process Habia

A short graduation can be achieved in two different ways. One way is to hold a section of hair vertically at a right angle or 90° to the scalp and position the hair that is to be cut between the fingers at an angle of around 45°.

An alternative way is to hold the hair horizontally from the scalp at a 45° angle and cut across the section following the shape of the head. Therefore, the 45° angle is achieved by either the position of the fingers or the position of the hair. You can see the step-by-step process for creating a short graduation in Chapter 6.

If the angle is greater or less than 45° the result of the graduation will change. If you use angles that are less than 45° the graduation will be minimal (almost like a one-length haircut). Where angles greater than 45° are used, the result will look more like a uniform layer.

When to use angles greater than 90°

Angles greater then 90° are used when you want to create a connected, layered look to incorporate hair lengths that vary from short to long. By directing the hair into angles greater than 90° you will be able to cut a greater range of lengths within the same haircut, and yet still enable the lengths to be blended together.

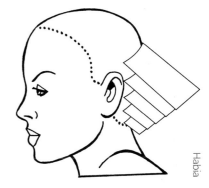

Holding hair horizontally for a graduated haircut

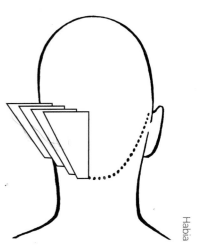

Holding hair vertically for a graduated haircut

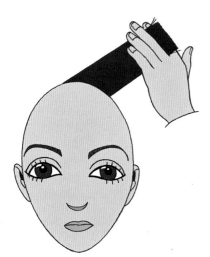

Hair that is overdirected can be used to blend long and short lengths together Habia

TIP	✔

It is important to be able to recognise when you need to increase the degree of the angle in a layered haircut, as failing to do so will result in the hair being cut too short.

CUTTING TECHNIQUES AND EFFECTS FOR HAIRDRESSING AND BARBERING

There are many different techniques that can be used to create a variety of looks. However, you must first perfect the basic techniques as these form the basis of the more advanced techniques that you will learn later.

The basic techniques are:

- club-cutting
- freehand techniques
- scissors over comb
- clipper over comb.

When you have mastered the basic techniques you can use them to develop the following cutting techniques and effects:

- graduating
- layering
- tapering
- thinning
- freehand cutting
- texturising
- using a razor.

As you progress through your career you will see how your cutting techniques change from the very basic, calculated and systematic cutting actions to those that can be described as individual, creative and innovative. These more adventurous techniques will eventually enable you to be even more creative and create looks that are known as avant-garde. This means you move from classic and current fashion haircuts to those that are amazingly creative, the forerunners of fashion.

Critical influencing factors that affect the choice of cutting technique

A critical influencing factor is an aspect about the client or their hair that will determine how you cut the hair and the look of the finished result. The critical influencing factors are identified during consultation with the client. Some factors are immediately visually apparent, some have to be tested for and others are identified by verbally communicating with your client.

The choice of cutting technique will be determined by the following factors:

- **The hair growth pattern** – all clients will have different hair growth patterns and you must be able to determine which cutting technique and cutting look will be most suitable. You need to remember that some hair growth patterns will restrict the look of the finished result.
- **The type of hair** – this means how straight, wavy or curly the hair is. Some clients may have hair that is too straight or too curly for a particular look, so you must be able to determine an appropriate cutting technique to achieve the desired result for the type of hair.
- **The texture of the hair** – this is the diameter of an individual strand of hair, i.e. how fine, medium or coarse the hair is. The texture of some client's hair may mean that you have to adapt your cutting techniques to achieve a particular look, or it may mean the texture of your client's hair is not suitable for a particular look.

- **The density of the hair** – this means the amount of hair on the head, i.e. how abundant or sparse the hair is. You may have to use a range of texturising techniques for clients with very abundant hair if you are to achieve a particular look. Likewise, you can make very sparse hair look thicker with some cutting techniques.

- **The look the client desires** – ensuring the style enhances the client's face shape and features and the shape of their head, as well as the shape of their body, is a critical factor of the consultation process. Some clients may dislike prominent features, which can be disguised with clever cutting and styling techniques.

- **The presence of male pattern baldness** – some men may have a particular pattern of baldness that they would like to disguise or that may affect your choice of techniques for cutting the hair.

- **The presence of added hair** – you need to be aware if the client has any hair extensions or hair pieces before the hair is cut. You must identify and use cutting techniques which will blend the added hair to the natural hair.

- **Hair elasticity** – the properties of elasticity within the hair change when the hair is wet or dry. Therefore you have to know if you should choose a cutting technique for wet hair or for dry hair.

You will find more detail about these factors that affect hair cutting in Chapter 2, Hair and Skin Structure and Analysis.

Using the cutting techniques and effects in hairdressing and barbering

By careful consultation with the client to identify their requirements, followed by the correct analysis of the characteristics of their hair, you can begin to determine the most appropriate cutting technique to achieve the desired result. You can cut hair using a number of different techniques and in many cases you will combine the cutting techniques, rather than using just one on an individual client.

Club-cutting

By using the club-cutting technique the hair length is reduced: the ends are cut to a blunt, even length, but the weight and bulk of the hair remain. Therefore, this technique is one that is common for many of the looks you will create. It is particularly good to use for creating straight, precision haircuts where the weight of the hair is required to be maintained. You need to be aware that cutting hair with this technique does restrict the amount of movement that can be created once the hair is styled because of the weight that remains at the ends of the hair.

The technique can be used on a wide range of different hair types and textures. This means that you can use this technique on hair that is straight, wavy or curly, on hair that is coarse, medium or fine in texture.

Club-cutting can be carried out when the hair is wet or dry, though a more precise and even result can be created on wet hair.

> **IT'S A FACT!**
>
> Club-cutting is very beneficial for fine hair, which can look more abundant if this technique is used.

Habia

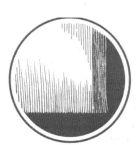

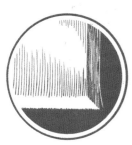

The result of club- and bevel cutting

Habia

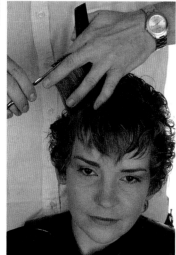

Club-cutting

You can club-cut hair using finely serrated and non-serrated scissors by holding the hair evenly between the fingers and then cutting the hair to the desired length. When club-cutting hair to very short lengths it is impossible to hold the hair between the fingers; therefore, you can hold the hair out at the required angle on a comb, and club-cut over the comb using either scissors or clippers. This technique is known as *scissors or clippers over comb*.

Summary for club-cutting

- Length of hair is reduced.
- Weight and bulk of the hair are retained.
- Can be carried out on wet or dry hair.
- Best technique for fine hair.
- Scissors or clippers can be used.

IT'S A FACT! !

If you hold the hair between your fingers as if you were going to club-cut, but then, rather than keeping the hair straight, turn the hair slightly to curl around your middle finger, the blades of the scissors will cut through the hair at a slight angle, creating a bevelled effect. The bevelled hair will allow the hair to curl a little more at the ends.

Freehand techniques

Freehand cutting techniques involve cutting without holding the hair with the hand, fingers or any tools, such as combs. Freehand cutting can be carried out with scissors or clippers and used for the following:

- cutting hair where there is a strong hair growth pattern;
- texturising hair to reduce bulk and length in certain areas;
- removing small amounts of individual hair;
- blending long and short lengths together;
- cutting the critical length of hair with a curl or wave movement;
- cutting an 'Afro' shape into African-type hair;
- creating patterns in hair.

Freehand cutting is very useful where you have a client with a very strong hair growth pattern at the fringe or nape area. For example, if your client has a cowlick, widow's peak or nape whorls, the hair will not lie straight, but in a variety of different directions. By allowing the hair to fall in its natural position before cutting, you can safely remove the unwanted length by using the tips of the scissors in a slicing or pointing action. This cutting technique prevents the removal of too much hair, or hair sticking out at an unwanted angle following the styling of a haircut.

Sometimes, on completion of a haircut and finish, you may notice that the hair is bulky or slightly too long in a particular area. The bulk and/or length can be removed using freehand a cutting technique known as *slicing*.

Slicing is carried out by inserting your open scissors at an angle to the length of hair then sliding the scissors down the length, while at the same time very gently, slightly, but not completely, closing the scissor blades together.

Freehand cutting can also be used to remove a small amount of stray hairs that may appear once the hair has been styled and dried following a haircut. This technique is excellent for cutting African-type hair into a natural 'Afro'-type hairstyle.

Using freehand cutting techniques also aids the prevention of cutting hair too short. For example, if you apply too much tension on wet curly or wavy hair during the haircut, once the hair is dry, the hair may be shorter than both you and your client expected. Therefore, if areas such as the hair at the fringe and nape areas or at the longest point of the haircut are cut using a freehand technique, without tension, you will eliminate the risk of the overall look being too short.

Blending very long to very short lengths can be achieved by using a freehand technique. Some haircuts may have a great deal of length at the nape of the neck, or the lengths at the back of the haircut, yet be quite short around the front hairline. By slicing from the short lengths through to the longer lengths you can achieve some form of connection in what may otherwise be an unintentionally disconnected haircut.

Clippers can be used using a freehand cutting technique in very creative ways. Patterns can be cut into the hair by using a template or stencil, or, for very artistic haircutters, by true freehand methods. The patterns can be two or three-dimensional. They can be pictorial, abstract or geometric designs. African-type hair is particularly suitable for this type of cutting, though designs can also be created on Asian and Caucasian hair. You can see some freehand clipper-cut designs in Chapter 6, the step by step by MK.

Clippers can also be used when carrying out freehand techniques on long hair. This is particularly useful if you want to create an interesting or alternative look to the front of a one-length bob. The hair can be combed into place and then the blades of the clippers can be used to create the shape of the front edges.

TIP

If you are slicing through hair to texturise or to remove unwanted bulk, it is important not to actually close the scissor blades together as you slice down the hair shaft, as you may remove too much hair.

ACTIVITY

Practise sliding the scissors through hair on a mannequin block before you try the technique on a client. See how far you can close the blades of the scissors together as you are sliding down the hair shaft without removing too much hair, or creating unwanted 'steps'.

TIP

The freehand technique can be carried out on wet or dry hair using scissors with a non-serrated edge. However, do take care to ensure the client's comfort if using slicing techniques on dry hair as this can pull and tear the hair if not done correctly.

IT'S A FACT!

Although freehand techniques are normally carried out with the use of hands, fingers, tools or other equipment to hold the hair, sometimes you may want to use a comb to lift and loosely hold the hair in place while freehand cutting the ends of the hair. This technique is particularly useful when freehand cutting near the face – as it prevents the scissors coming dangerously close to the eyes.

Summary for freehand cutting

● Useful where there is a strong hair growth pattern at the nape or the fringe area.

● The length and weight of the hair can be reduced at the same time.

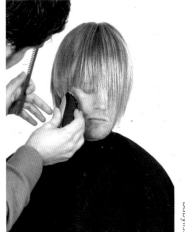

BaByliss

Clippers can be used to create the outline of a haircut

- Can be used to remove unwanted bulk to a finished look.
- Good technique for removing small amounts of stray hairs.
- Can be used on a variety of hair types and textures.
- Can be used to create patterns in hair.
- Useful technique to ensure that curly or wavy hair is not cut too short.

Scissors over comb

This technique is more often used in barbering, though it is also used in ladies' hairdressing where the hair length is required to be cut shorter than would be possible if you were using your fingers to hold the hair in position. Scissors over comb is usually used to create a graduated look on very short hair by lifting the hair with a comb and holding the hair at the required angle before cutting to remove unwanted length. On very short hair a soft, pliable comb with fine teeth can be used to hold the hair; however, when cutting coarse or abundant hair a wide-toothed comb can be used to prevent client discomfort. The technique can be carried out on wet or dry hair.

TIP

When cutting hair using the scissors over comb technique you should ensure that you have 'fast scissors and slow comb'. This means that as you move the comb up the head, your scissors should open and close quickly to cut the hair as you move the comb through the hair. If you open and close the scissors too slowly you will create steps in the finished haircut.

TIP

Some hairdressers and barbers use the tips of the scissors to lift the hair into place over the comb before cutting – if you do this, ensure that the scissors are closed to prevent cutting the hair as you lift it into place.

ACTIVITY

You can practise the action of cutting with scissors over the comb before you do it on a client. Try holding your scissors vertically in front of you, in a horizontal line, with scissors in front of the comb. Then, as you lift the comb in an upward movement, open and close the scissors at the same time as the comb is lifted. You have to be sure that the comb is lifted at the same rate of time as the scissors to ensure that the comb is always in line with the scissors.

Summary for scissors over comb cutting

- Often used in barbering.
- Best technique for cutting hair to very short lengths.
- Can be used on a variety of different hair types and textures.

Clipper over comb

Clippers can be used over a comb to create looks similar to those created by scissors over comb. This technique, which should be carried out on dry hair, is particularly useful when cutting hair to very short lengths as it is more efficient than using scissors, as the blades of clippers pass over each other the hair is cut much quicker.

Summary for clipper over comb cutting

- Quick and efficient way of cutting hair in very short layers.
- Best carried out on dry hair as this use of clippers can pull and tear wet hair.

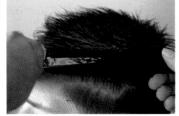

Scissor over comb

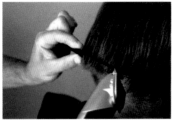

Clipper over comb

Graduation

The word *graduation* is used to describe hair that has been cut at a variety of angles to create different lengths within the same haircut. Graduation can be long graduation or short graduation. The type of graduation is determined where the longer or shorter lengths of hair start and finish on the interior or exterior of the haircut.

Sometimes the interior of the haircut is shorter than the exterior. This is usually known as a *long graduation*. When the interior of a haircut is longer than the exterior, it is known as a *short graduation*.

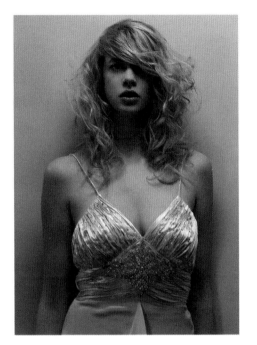

Long Graduation Hair by the Nikki Froud Artistic Team; products by Clynol

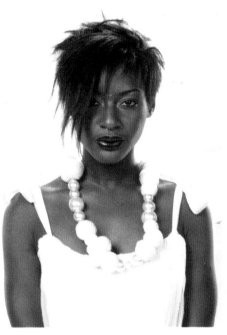

Short graduation Hair by Anne Veck for Anne Veck Hair; photography by David Howard

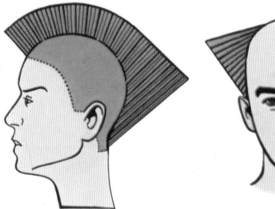

Long and short graduation cutting projections Habia

> **IT'S A FACT** !
>
> Many hairdressers call a one-length 'bob' a reverse graduation. This is because, on certain one-length bobs, the hair is sometimes cut so that each section is slightly longer than the previous section. The slightly longer layers can look as though they have a very small degree of graduation in them on the underside of the haircut. The longer lengths are able to turn under the shorter hair, helping the finished result to have a classic 'turned-under' bob look.

Graduation can be carried out by using scissors, clippers or razors on wet or dry hair. However, razors should only be used on wet hair and clippers are best used on hair that is dry.

Summary of graduation cutting

- A technique used to blend a range of different hair lengths together.
- Can be used on a variety of different hair types and textures to create a wide range of hairstyles and looks.
- Graduation can be created by using scissors, clippers or razors.

Layering

Layering is a generic term that describes hair that is cut to a variety of lengths, which can be very short or very long, where the layers can be connected together or can be disconnected.

Layering can also refer to hair that is graduated. A graduated haircut can have a short interior and a longer exterior length, or the hair can be left longer on the interior and have a shorter exterior length. Alternatively layered hair can be all the same length, a uniform length. This is generally known as a *uniform or basic layered haircut*. Here the hair is cut into lengths that are exactly the same over the head. The hair can be very short or very long, but the length of the layers will always be the same.

Graduated and uniform layered haircuts will have layers that blend together to form a connected haircut. However, sometimes a layered look can be created where the layers do not connect together. This is known as a *disconnected haircut*. Disconnected haircuts require a great deal of skill and are usually used to demonstrate the more creative and innovative effects of haircutting.

Layers can be created using scissors, clippers or razors and can be carried out on hair that is wet or dry.

> **TIP** ✔
>
> A disconnected haircut must still have an overall coherent look, but as you will not be able to cross-check the cut in the same way a connected cut is checked, you must look at the finished cut to ensure the cut is aesthetically pleasing.

Summary for layering

- Technique can be used on any hair type, texture or length.
- Can be cut using scissors, clippers and razors.
- Can create a wide range of looks.
- The layers can be connected or disconnected.
- The layers can graduate, or be uniform in length.

Tapering

When you are tapering hair you can reduce both the length and weight of hair at the same time. The technique can be carried out in a variety of ways with scissors, clippers and razors on wet or dry hair.

The overall result of tapering will leave the hair finer at the ends than the roots. Too much weight at the ends of hair can make it more difficult to create interest in the final styling as the weight of the hair makes it more likely to be straighter and flatter. Therefore, the removal of weight at the ends of the hair will encourage movement, as the different lengths of hair will curl more easily.

There are several ways to taper hair:

- **Tapering with scissors** – If tapering with scissors, the cutting action will be one of sliding the scissors, using a backwards and forward movement on the lower one third of the hair length from the points to the roots and back again. The scissors are inserted into the section to be cut and as the cutting action takes place, the blades very slightly and gently close together. However, you must not close the blades completely, or you will remove too much hair. This type of tapering can only be carried out on dry hair. If you use this cutting action when the hair is wet, the strands will stick together resulting in an uneven and choppy look.

- **Back-combing tapering** – You can also use your scissors to taper hair using a backcombing technique. You can only do this on dry hair. In the area you wish to taper, take a small section of hair and with a wide-toothed comb, gently and loosely backcomb some of the section towards the root. Then, on the remaining hair, use the sliding action to reduce the length and weight. Once you have removed the backcombing at the root area, you will have a tapered, texturised section with a variety of hair lengths within it.

- **Tapering with clippers** – Tapering can also be carried out on dry hair with clippers. A small section of hair can be loosely twisted and then, using small clippers, skim the outside of the twist gently with the clipper blades, moving the clippers from the last third of the section to the points of the hair. If you are using this method, it is important not to place the clippers directly into the twisted section, or you will remove too much hair.

  Alternatively you can use this twisting technique and insert the points of scissors into the twist at various places between the last third of the hair length and the points of the hair.

- **Tapering with a razor** – The hair must be wet for this technique. The razor is inserted at a shallow angle on the last third of the section and gently skims along the hair shaft towards the points. You can do this on top of the section, or underneath it. Do not insert the razor at an angle more than 45° as this will result in the removal of too much hair.

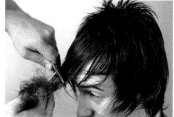

Insertion of razor into hair

Summary for tapering

- These techniques are used to reduce the length and weight of the hair simultaneously.
- They are only carried out on dry hair, unless you are using the razor tapering technique.
- Scissors, clippers and razors can be used.
- Encourages curl and movement in hair.

Thinning

Thinning is a method of reducing the weight of hair while maintaining the length. It is normally carried out on abundant and coarser hair that is often bushy and difficult to style. You can use scissors, thinning scissors, razors or clippers to thin hair.

Habia

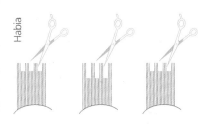

Pointing insertion patterns

Habia

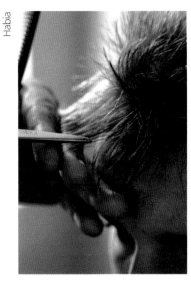

Pointing hair

There are several tools that you can use to thin hair:

- **Using scissors to thin hair** – The scissors can be used to thin hair using a 'pointing' technique. This can be carried out when the hair is wet or dry. It is achieved by taking a section of hair that you wish to thin and inserting the tips of the scissors into the section to remove some of the hair at intervals across the section. The more hair that is pointed out, the finer the ends of the hair will be. It is best to do this on the last one third of the hair section, unless you are trying to create a really drastic or avant-garde effect when you intentionally want to have very short lengths at the root section. If you do cut it close to the roots, you may find areas of hair that stick out during the styling of the haircut.

A variation of the pointing technique can be slicing. This is best carried out when the hair is dry with non-serrated scissors. A section of hair is held between the fingers and the scissors are used to slice through the free ends of the section. This is achieved by inserting the open scissors into the hair section and then, gently, slightly closing the scissors as they move towards the ends of the hair. Do not close the scissors completely, or you will create steps in the haircut. The advantage of the slicing technique over pointing is that the thinned hair is more blended and less choppy.

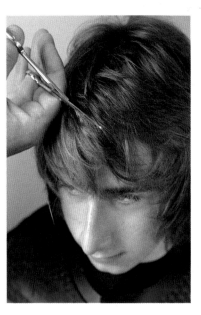

Slicing layered hair Habia

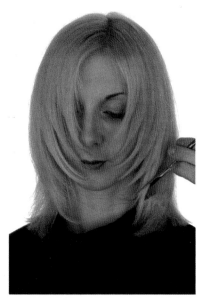

Slicing the perimeter of hair to create texture Habia

- **Using thinning scissors to thin hair** – Specially designed thinning scissors, which are also known as aesculap scissors or texturising scissors, can be used to thin the hair. These come in a range of different blade lengths and serration. You can learn about the different types of thinning scissors in Chapter 4, Tools, Equipment and Products. The thinning scissors have gaps in the cutting edge of the blades, which means that as the blades are closed, some of the hair remains uncut.

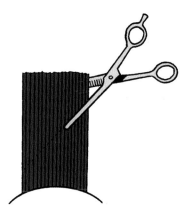

Insertion pattern for thinning hair Habia

Summary for thinning hair

- A method of reducing the weight without reducing the length of the hair.
- Can be carried out using scissors, clipper, thinning scissors and razors.

Texturising

The word *texturising* is a generic term used to describe the way a basic haircut, which looks very solid, can be 'broken up' or 'shattered' to create a range of different lengths within the original haircut, thus creating interest and movement, personalising the finished look and style.

Texturising is not the same as thinning. Thinning hair will reduce the bulk or weight and not length, whereas texturising can be used in a more flexible way. With texturising you can remove both the weight and the length, or just the weight. Texturising can take place on any area of a haircut. Fringes and solid lines can be softened, weight can be removed and shorter lengths can be cut to support longer lengths of hair. Texturising can be used within connected haircuts, but if used extensively can be used to create disconnected haircuts.

Texturising can be carried out on the ends of the hair, or in some cases, right through from the roots to the points. It can be completed during the haircut, or at the end of the haircut and style to individualise the cut for the client's specific requirements.

Pointing, slicing, slithering, chopping, channelling, weaving and chipping are just some of the names that are used to describe texturising techniques. In addition to these names many leading hairdressers who create innovative cutting techniques often have their own terminology for the individual texturising techniques that they use.

Texturising can be carried out on all hair types and textures. Even fine, sparse hair can look fuller with a calculated amount of texturising.

Texturising can be carried out with scissors, clippers and razors.

Summary for texturising hair

- A technique used to remove weight and/or length from hair.
- Individualised techniques adapted for the client's specific requirements can be achieved through texturising.
- Can be carried out in a variety of ways on hair types and textures.

Summary of cutting techniques

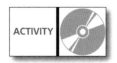

ACTIVITY

Effects of cutting
techniques

Technique	Reduce length	Reduce weight
Club-cutting	yes	no
Freehand	yes	yes
Scissors/clippers over comb	yes	no
Tapering	yes	yes
Thinning	no	yes
Texturising	yes	yes

CREATING CUTTING LOOKS

What is meant by the term *cutting look*? It means the overall finished hairstyle that is achieved from the haircut.

All hairstyling relies on a good foundation – that of the haircut. Without it, the hairstyle cannot be achieved. Cutting can therefore be said to be one of the most crucial aspects of hairdressing and barbering.

The looks for hairdressing and barbering are:

- one-length looks
- uniform layered looks
- graduated looks on long and short hair
- looks that include a fringe
- classic looks for hairdressing and traditional looks for barbering
- current looks
- emerging fashion looks.

One-length looks

A basic one-length cut is created by first cutting a base or guideline to the length that the client requests, and then ensuring that each subsequent section is cut to meet the length of the first guideline. You can read and see how a one-length cut is created in Chapter 6, Step by Step.

With this haircut there is one, overall, even and level outside length to the finished look. The length of a one-length haircut can vary from chin length to well below the shoulders.

The term *bob cut* is one that is often associated with a one-length look. In Chapter 1, Cutting Philosophy, you learnt about the creativity of Vidal Sassoon when he cut the first bob shapes in the 1960s. These were a complete change from other hair fashions of the time. That classic shape still remains today, but the one-length look has changed and adapted over the years to become the more individualised look we have today. Today's one-length looks are created using a combination of different cutting techniques from club-cutting to texturing. The use of club-cutting ensures a neat, precision edge to the haircut, whereas texturising can soften the line and add interest and movement to the overall shape.

The outside edge of the one-length look can vary. The look can be horizontally straight with a square, even outline, or the outside line can be angled towards or away from the face. The shape of neckline can also be changed to create a variety of looks. The neckline can be horizontal, symmetric, asymmetric, angular or curved.

The fringe is another way in which one-length haircuts can be altered to suit the individual client requirements. You can adapt the fringe shape to suit different-shaped faces. For example, if your client has a long face, a heavy fringe can shorten the look of the face. For rectangular-shaped faces, a curved or rounded fringe shape can soften hard, angular looks. However, a curved heavy fringe would not be suitable for round faces, as the fringe would shorten the face and accentuate the roundness of the face.

Uniform layered looks

A uniform layered look is one in which the lengths of the layers are of an even, uniform length throughout the haircut. A uniform haircut can be very short, or very long. An extreme example of this would be hair that has been cut by clippers using a clipper guide to a length of 9 mm. The hair will be very short, but it will also be a uniform length of 9 mm throughout.

One of the most crucial aspects for creating a uniform layered haircut is to ensure that the hair is held at a 90° angle to the scalp and cut to the same length all over the head, remembering to follow the contours of the head shape. If you change the angle in which the hair is held, the shape will not be in uniform layers, but graduated layers.

In reality very few haircuts are a uniform layer throughout. Most layered haircuts are a combination of graduation and uniform layers.

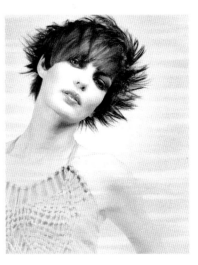

Sean Hanna

Graduated looks on long and short hair

Graduated is the term that is used to describe a hairstyle that gradually changes in length from long to short or short to long. Sometimes the degree of graduation can be very high. For example, hair may be quite short on the interior of the haircut, but increase in length to below the shoulders on the exterior of the haircut. Graduation may be quite subtle, in which case the haircut almost looks like a uniform layer.

Graduation can be achieved in the haircut by slightly increasing or decreasing the lengths of the sections you are cutting as you move through the haircut. This is normally achieved by using cutting angles of around 45°. If the degree of graduation is very high, which means the lengths of the hair

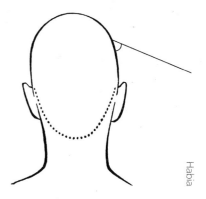

45° angle

Habia

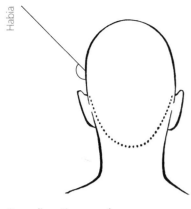

Habia

Overdirection angle

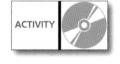

ACTIVITY

Identify the fringe shaper

go from very short to very long and there is likely to be big difference in the lengths of the layers, you would have to *overdirect* the hair – hold it at an angle greater than 90°. Overdirection is very useful when you want a connected, but long graduation.

Looks that include fringes

Fringes are an important part of any haircut and can change the whole look for the client. Sometimes, just cutting a fringe into an existing haircut can make the client feel as though they have had a complete restyle.

Fringes can be:

- long
- short
- straight
- curved

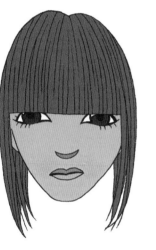

Long fringe Habia

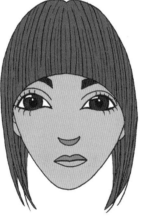

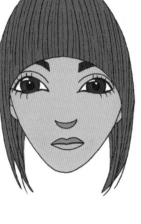

Curved fringe Habia

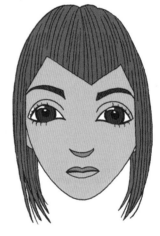

Angular fringe Habia

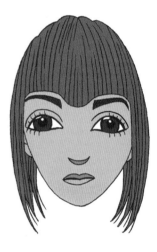

Symmetric fringe Habia

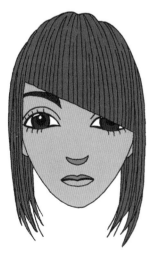

Asymmetric fringe Habia

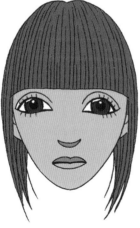

Heavy fringe Habia

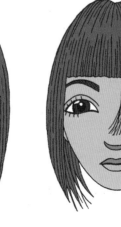

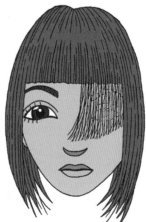

Double fringe Habia

Textured fringe Habia

- angular
- symmetric
- asymmetric
- heavy
- fine
- texturised
- double
- textured.

When cutting a fringe it is very important to consider the following:

- type of hair
- texture of hair
- hair growth patterns
- shape of the client's face
- recession areas.

Type of hair to be considered when cutting fringes

You need to remember that while curly or wavy hair may look straight and of a particular length when it is wet, it will look shorter and curlier when it is dry. Therefore, you must take great care to allow for the natural movement of the hair to prevent the fringe looking too short.

It is important to ensure that the fringe your client chooses is suitable for their hair type. For example, if the client would like a geometric, angular-shaped fringe, which relies on straight precision cutting, then only absolutely straight hair will allow such a precise, finished result.

Texture of hair to be considered when cutting fringes

If the hair is very coarse you may have to texturise the fringe area to prevent it looking too bulky. Fine hair may need to be club-cut if you want the fringe to have an impact on the overall result of the finished hairstyle. The texture of hair can also play an important part in changing the apparent shape of the face. For example, if a client wanted a fringe, but had a round or square face and also had coarse, heavy hair, it would shorten the appearance of the face even more. However, by clever and careful cutting techniques, including texturising to reduce the weight but not the length, the fringe can be cut, while at the same time allowing the forehead to be seen through the hair, thus increasing the apparent length of the face.

Hair growth patterns to be considered when cutting fringes

Hair that does not have an adverse hair growth pattern will grow straight down at the front hairline. This means that you can safely cut a fringe that will lie flat and even. However, most clients will have some hair that grows in a particular direction, however slight, and this must be taken into consideration. The most common hair growth patterns are cowlicks and widow's peaks.

A cowlick is a hair growth pattern in which the hair grows back from the front hairline. Many can be semi-circular in shape and off-centre, others are just a slight change in direction of hair growth. However, in very extreme cases, the hairline at the front of the head can grow back from one side to the other, making it impossible to have any sort of fringe. Sometimes, a client may have two cowlicks at the front hairline that converge together in the middle of the forehead, making a point in the middle of the fringe area. This is known as a widow's peak. Widow's peaks can also be hair that grows back from a point in the middle of the forehead. All of these hair growth patterns are critical factors that must be considered when cutting hair at the front hairline. You can read more about hair growth patterns in Chapter 2, Hair and Skin Structure and Analysis.

As a hairdresser or barber, you have to make a decision based on your analysis of the direction of hair growth. With a very slight hair growth pattern in one direction or another, a full fringe can be cut. However, if the growth is stronger, you may want to leave the hair longer, or work with the direction of hair growth to make a texturised fringe that does not rely on sitting flat and straight.

Shape of the client's face to be considered when cutting fringes

The shape and length of the fringe can drastically alter the apparent shape of the client's face. In fact, cutting a fringe is one of the best methods for reducing the appearance of an overlong face, or softening hard, angular features.

The facial shape that is considered to be perfect is an oval face. This means that the face is evenly balanced with the overall appearance likened to the shape of an egg. The forehead will be slightly wider than the chin. The length of the face will be slightly longer than the width. The jawline will be slightly curved, but not angular. Therefore, if the face is longer or wider than oval, the hair can be used to enhance the facial shape by making it appear more oval than it really is.

A heavy fringe can be used to shorten the length of a face. Angular bone structures can be softened with a rounded, soft, texturised fringe. Clients with round faces who request a full fringe could have a fine texturised fringe in which the forehead can still be seen slightly through the hair. This means the client will be pleased that they have a fringe, yet, because the fringe has been texturised, it does not shorten the appearance of the length of the face.

Recession areas to be considered when cutting fringes

Recession areas are normally found at the temporal regions of the forehead. Men are more likely to have recession area, but some women do too.

Habia

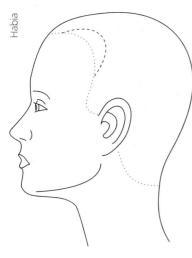

Recession area

Fringes are a good way to disguise a recession area, and men who have some male pattern baldness may intentionally grow their hair longer in such places. Therefore, ensure the consultation you carry out with the client identifies if they wish to leave their hair longer in these areas.

You also have to consider the distance between the eyebrows and the hairline in order to identify if the client has a high or low hairline pattern. Clients with a low hairline growth pattern will have little space between the eyebrows and the hairline. This means that full, heavy fringes should be avoided. Some clients may have very high hairlines. In these cases, a fringe can disguise a prominent forehead.

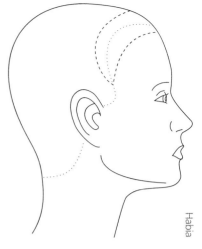

Habia

High and low hair growth patterns

Classic looks

The term *classic look* is used to describe a hairstyle that is timeless and often elegant. Classic looks are haircuts and styles that have stood the test of time and are created over and over again, year after year. It is often the more basic cutting techniques and effects that are considered to be classic shapes, for example, the one-length bob, graduated and layered looks.

For a look to be 'classic' it does not have to look exactly the same each time it is created. Instead, the same basic shape can be created with a twist of individuality to update and refresh the look that has preceded it.

Traditional looks

This is the term used in barbering to describe timeless cutting looks.

Current looks

This is the term that is used to describe what is actually fashionable at the present time. Of course, current looks will constantly change. Hairdressing and barbering are industries which never stay the same. Each month and in every season and year a new style is created or a classic look is reinvented. The media – through television, magazines and cinema – can influence current looks. There are many haircuts that are created for clients because they have seen an actor or actress, or football player or soap star wearing a particular look.

Emerging fashion looks

Emerging fashion is the term that is given to looks that are created by hairdressers and barbers who are creative enough to experiment with different techniques. The techniques they investigate can lead to haircuts

> **TIP** ✔
>
> Be aware that when a client asks for a current look that is associated with a celebrity, you must be able to adapt it so that it is suitable for the individual characteristics of your client's face shape, hair type and texture.

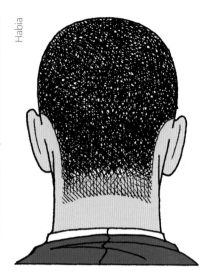

Tapered neckline

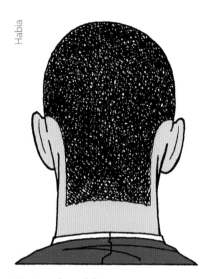

Squared neckline

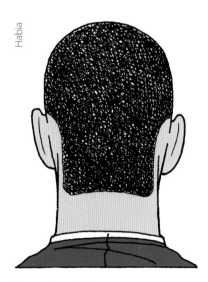

Round neckline

that may or may not turn into current or classic looks. However, whether a look is copied and becomes everyday fashion is not necessarily important. The significant thing is that the hairdresser or barber has had the courage to experiment and influence the industry. Being able to experiment can only happen once you have mastered the basic techniques for haircutting and practised until you feel confident enough to try new ideas.

Neckline shapes

The shape of the neckline can be as important as the shape of the rest of the haircut. Neckline shapes must be carefully considered when cutting hair very short – either on a man or a woman.

One of the most critical influencing factors that should be considered when cutting the neckline shape is the direction of hair growth. A neckline where there are no adverse hair growth patterns will have hair that grows flat and lies neatly at the nape of the neck. However, most clients do not have a nape hairline like this. The majority of clients will have hair that grows in one, two or even three different directions in whorls at the nape of the neck. Sometimes the hair grows to the centre, others it grows from the centre towards the front.

Neckline shapes for men

You must be very careful when cutting a neckline shape on a male client as some necklines can look feminine.

There are three traditional neckline shapes for male clients:

- tapered
- squared
- rounded.

Tapered A tapered neckline is one in which the hair is gradually blended from the neckline into the main body of the haircut. Sometimes, this can mean the hair is so short on the outer edge that it is almost invisible. The perimeter line will be soft, and not necessarily defined by a neat edge.

Squared This is a very masculine shape and although the shape is mainly used in barbering, it can also be used for female clients if an angular look is required. It is created by a straight vertical line that runs from behind the ears to the lower hairline. The lower hairline shape will be very straight and well defined.

Rounded This shape is more feminine, but can also be used for male clients. The neckline will have a gentle curve which runs around the hairline from ear to ear.

CROSS-CHECKING THE HAIRCUT

When you have completed your haircut using the required technique for the client's individual requirements, you must then check your work to ensure the cut has been carried out accurately. This is done by a process known as *cross-checking*. Everyone, no matter how experienced a hairdresser or barber they may be, should check their work on completion of the haircut. Not only does this ensure that the haircut is correct, but it also shows your client that you are proud of the quality of your work and care about the service you are providing.

Cross-checking can be carried out in two different ways:

- by holding the hair at a variety of angles and positions, therefore carrying out a physical cross-check;
- by visual means – looking at the finished result.

> **TIP**
>
> For total accuracy, cross-check the haircut when the hair is dried and styled as well as on completion of the haircut when the hair is still wet.

How to cross-check a layered haircut

If you have cut a uniform layer, this means that the hair is exactly the same length all over the client's head. So, cross-checking is very straightforward. By holding the hair at a right angle to the head and comparing the look and the shape of the layers, you should be able to see that the hair length is even throughout the head. You should not see longer lengths, stray hairs or unusual angles. Each section of cross-checked hair should be the same length as the previous section.

However, there are some exceptions to this. If the haircut is a mixture of uniform and graduated layers, you must remember this during the cross-check and ensure that the graduation aspect of the haircut blends accurately with the uniform length layers.

Another exception is where you have cut square layers. Square layers are used to create weight and interest in what otherwise would be a very basic layered haircut. When cross-checking square layers, you must allow for a more angular outline to the haircut that would not be visible in a basic uniform layer.

How to cross-check a graduated haircut

The best method for cross-checking a short graduated haircut is to check the hair lengths in the opposite way in which they have been cut.

For example, if you have used vertical sections to create the graduation, check the haircut by holding the hair in horizontal sections. If you horizontally held the hair at 45° during the graduation, use vertical cross-checking sections to ensure the angle of graduation is accurate.

The cross-check should confirm that there are no stray hairs and that the length and graduation of the hair follow the appropriate contours of the head to give an aesthetically pleasing and balanced result.

How to cross-check a one-length haircut

Although a one-length haircut may only have one line to check, it is crucial that the haircut is accurate, or the whole look will be unbalanced and unacceptable for the client.

To cross-check a one-length look you can hold the hair on opposite sides of the haircut and visually check that they are balanced. Another way you can do this, but which requires good coordination, is to run your fingers down two parts of the haircut at the same time. Place your fingers at the top of a section of the haircut and run your fingers down the hair length together. Make sure that you do this at the same speed with both hands, or you may get an incorrect result.

How to visually cross-check a haircut

Even if you are satisfied with the physical cross-check, you must also visually check that the haircut is balanced and complements the client's head and facial shape.

You can visually cross-check the haircut by standing back away from the client and looking at the cut centrally and then from a variety of different directions. During the visual check, lift the hair and allow it to fall back into the shape that it will be styled.

Ask yourself the following questions:

- Does the hair fall evenly and balanced?
- Is the weight line of the haircut in the correct place?
- Does each side of the haircut look even, or, in the case of an asymmetric haircut, aesthetically pleasing?

Making changes after the cross-check

It is important for you to recognise when you need to correct a haircut following the cross-check. If, after holding the hair you find lengths, angles or weight that you were not expecting to find, check why they are there before you cut them off. If you just cut the hair without investigating why the 'fault' is there, you may change the entire shape of the haircut without realising.

The end of the cross-check, both physical and visual, provides the perfect opportunity to 'individualise' a haircut. This means that following the completion of the haircut, you may see scope to create a look or finish to the haircut that you did not plan with the client at the consultation. For example, you may find that the fringe shape looks heavier than you planned and would look better if the weight was removed by slicing through the ends. However, always consult with the client before making any changes.

SERVICES TO ENHANCE THE HAIRCUT

Providing you have cut the hair using techniques that are appropriate for the client's hair type, texture and density, the styling should be easy for the client to manage.

Without a good basic shape it would be impossible to create a good hairstyle. Once the haircut and finish is complete you should demonstrate to the client how they should style their hair at home. At this stage you should also recommend and demonstrate how to use the styling products that will support and maintain the look. In addition make a recommendation about when the client should return to the salon for the next haircut. Remember that hair grows on average 1.25 cm each month. Therefore, if the hair cut is short and precision cut, the client should have their hair cut again within six weeks.

Colouring is a major salon service and almost every haircut can be enhanced by the use of colour. The colour can be used to define the haircut shape. Darker colours can be used to create a denser, more solid appearance, whereas lighter colours can be used to highlight and add interest to selected areas of the haircut. With colour you can literally paint the haircut.

Some clients may need to have a little style support to enhance a particular haircut, especially if their hair if fine or sparse. Today's perming techniques are not at all harsh; many are semi-permanent, but they will enable the client to maintain their haircut between salon visits.

Assessment of knowledge and understanding

Test yourself on the content of this chapter by answering these questions.

Assessment activity level A

Match the correct definition of the cutting techniques by drawing a line between the boxes.

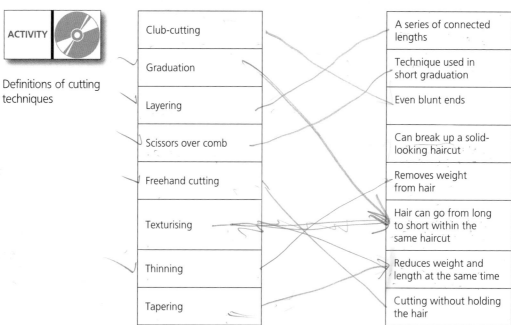

ACTIVITY

Definitions of cutting techniques

Cutting technique	Definition
Club-cutting	A series of connected lengths
Graduation	Technique used in short graduation
Layering	Even blunt ends
Scissors over comb	Can break up a solid-looking haircut
Freehand cutting	Removes weight from hair
Texturising	Hair can go from long to short within the same haircut
Thinning	Reduces weight and length at the same time
Tapering	Cutting without holding the hair

The answer to this activity can be found at the end of the book.

Assessment activity level A

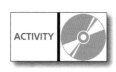

ACTIVITY

Fill in the blanks

Answer the following questions by writing in the missing word from the list below.

1 It is important for you to recognise when you need to _Collect_ a haircut following the cross-check.

2 One of the most critical influencing factors that should be considered when cutting the neckline shape is the direction of hair _growth_

3 Sometimes a layered look can be created where the layers do not connect together. This is known as a _disconnect_ haircut.

4 One of the most crucial aspects for creating a uniform layered haircut is to ensure that the hair is held at a _right angle_ to the scalp and cut to the same length all over the head, remembering to following the contours of the head shape.

5 You also have to consider the distance between the eyebrows and the _forehead_ in order to identify of the client has a high or low hairline pattern.

hair line

6 With a _texturing_ technique, fringes and solid lines can be softened, weight can be removed and shorter lengths can be cut to support longer lengths of hair.

7 _Freehand_ cutting techniques refer to a cut that is made without holding the hair with either the hand, fingers or other tools, such as combs.

8 A _Cowlick_ is a hair growth pattern in which the hair grows back from the front hairline.

9 It is important to ensure that the fringe your client chooses is suitable for their hair _type_.

10 _forty five degree_ angles are used during short graduation.

disconnected	hairline	type	cowlick	texturing
correct	right angle	freehand	growth	forty five-degree

The answers to this activity can be found at the end of the book.

Assessment activity level B

Select the correct answer below.

1 Club-cutting results in:

  a hair cut to uneven lengths
  b hair cut to even lengths
  c hair more likely to be curly
  d short hair

2 Hair type is:

  a how coarse the hair is
  b how fine the hair is
  c how curly the hair is
  d how dense the hair is

3 Slicing hair used when texturising on dry hair should be carried out using:

  a thinning scissors
  b non-serrated scissors
  c serrated scissors
  d clippers

4 Cutting hair without holding it is known as:

  a club-cutting
  b thinning
  c texturising
  d freehand cutting

5 Too much tension applied to wet hair during cutting will result in:

  a bulky hair
  b short too short

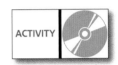

ACTIVITY

Multiple choice

c hair too long
d straight hair

6 Hair can be cut to a guaranteed length with clippers by using:

a fingers
b comb
c scissors
d guides *(circled)*

7 Layered hair can be:

a disconnected *(circled)*
b curly
c wavy
d natural

8 A cowlick will prevent a fringe:

a being too long
b being too short *(circled)*
c being cut
d lying flat *(circled)*

9 A face that is rectangular in shape will be:

a short and round
b short and angular
c long and angular
d long and round

10 A recession area can be found at the:

a nape
b crown
c temples *(circled)*
d sides

The answers to this activity can be found at the end of the book.

Assessment activity level C

club - cutting

1 Name a cutting technique that can make fine hair look thicker.
2 What is significant about a freehand cutting technique? *The hair is held without hand, and tools*
3 How can bevelled effects be created? *by curling the hair between the*
4 Why is it important not to close the scissor blades together when *fingers* using a slicing technique? *before c*
5 What is the purpose of using clipper guides?
6 What is another name for a reverse graduation? *bob,*
7 What is the result of tapering?
8 What is the result of thinning hair?
9 What is emerging fashion?
10 Name two different neckline shapes.

The answers to this activity can be found at the end of the book.

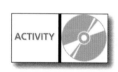

ACTIVITY

Multiple choice

to creat a guaranteed even length for the haircut

Assessment activity levels A and B: Word search

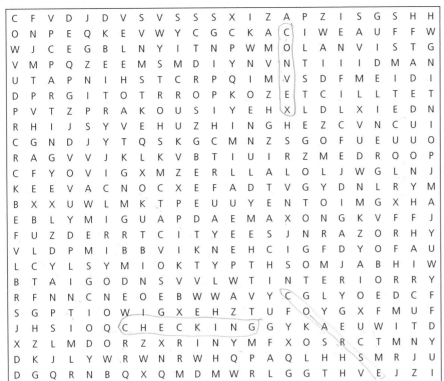

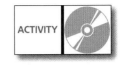

Word search

C	F	V	D	J	D	V	S	V	S	S	S	X	I	Z	A	P	Z	I	S	G	S	H	H
O	N	P	E	Q	K	E	V	W	Y	C	G	C	K	A	C	I	W	E	A	U	F	F	W
W	J	C	E	G	B	L	N	Y	I	T	N	P	W	M	O	L	A	N	V	I	S	T	G
V	M	P	Q	Z	E	E	M	S	M	D	I	Y	N	V	N	T	I	I	I	D	M	A	N
U	T	A	P	N	I	H	S	T	C	R	P	Q	I	M	V	S	D	F	M	E	I	D	I
D	P	R	G	I	T	O	T	R	R	O	P	K	O	Z	E	T	C	I	L	L	T	E	T
P	V	T	Z	P	R	A	K	O	U	S	I	Y	E	H	X	L	D	L	X	I	E	D	N
R	H	I	J	S	Y	V	E	H	U	Z	H	I	N	G	H	E	Z	C	V	N	C	U	I
C	G	N	D	J	Y	T	Q	S	K	G	C	M	N	Z	S	G	O	F	U	E	U	U	O
R	A	G	V	V	J	K	L	K	V	B	T	I	U	I	R	Z	M	E	D	R	O	O	P
C	F	Y	O	V	I	G	X	M	Z	E	R	L	L	A	L	O	L	J	W	G	L	N	J
K	E	E	V	A	C	N	O	C	X	E	F	A	D	T	V	G	Y	D	N	L	R	Y	M
B	X	X	U	W	L	M	K	T	P	E	U	U	Y	E	N	T	O	I	M	G	X	H	A
E	B	L	Y	M	I	G	U	A	P	D	A	E	M	A	X	O	N	G	K	V	F	F	J
F	U	Z	D	E	R	R	T	C	I	T	Y	E	E	S	J	N	R	A	Z	O	R	H	Y
V	L	D	P	M	I	B	B	V	I	K	N	E	H	C	I	G	F	D	Y	O	F	A	U
L	C	Y	L	S	Y	M	I	O	K	T	Y	P	T	H	S	O	M	J	A	B	H	I	W
B	T	A	I	G	O	D	N	S	V	V	L	W	T	I	N	T	E	R	I	O	R	R	Y
R	F	N	N	C	N	E	O	E	B	W	W	A	V	Y	C	G	L	Y	O	E	D	C	F
S	G	P	T	I	O	W	I	G	X	E	H	Z	T	U	F	O	Y	G	X	F	M	U	F
J	H	S	I	O	Q	C	H	E	C	K	I	N	G	G	Y	K	A	E	U	W	I	T	D
X	Z	L	M	D	O	R	Z	X	R	I	N	Y	M	F	X	O	S	R	C	T	M	N	Y
D	K	J	L	Y	W	R	W	N	R	W	H	Q	P	A	Q	L	H	H	S	M	R	J	U
D	G	Q	R	N	B	Q	X	Q	M	D	M	W	R	L	G	G	T	H	V	E	J	Z	I

angle	checking	chipping	club	coarse
comb	concave	convex	curly	fine
graduation	guideline	haircut	individualised	interior
length	movement	parting	pointing	root
razor	scissors	short	tapering	texturising
thinning	type	uniform	wavy	

The answers to this activity can be found at the end of the book.

CUTTING TECHNIQUES H6/H7/H21/H22/H27

Assessment activity level C: Crossword

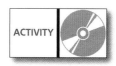

ACTIVITY

Crossword

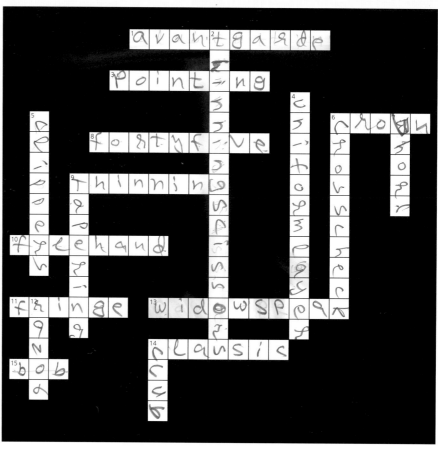

avant garde

Across
1. A look that is a forerunner of fashion (two words)
3. Cutting method used to texturise
6. A double one of these makes the hair difficult to cut
8. Angle commonly used during graduation (two words)
9. Technique that reduces weight but not length
10. You do not hold the hair with this technique
11. Covers the forehead
13. Hair growth pattern found at the front hairline (two words)
14. This look is timeless
15. One-length hair cut

Down
2. Tool used to remove weight from the hair (two words)
4. A ninety-degree angle is used during this type of haircut (two words)
5. You can use these over a comb
6. Used to ensure the haircut is correct (two words)
7. Hair growth pattern found in the nape
9. Reduces length and weight at the same time
12. Only use on wet hair
14. Cutting technique which produces blunt ends

The answers to this activity can be found at the end of the book.

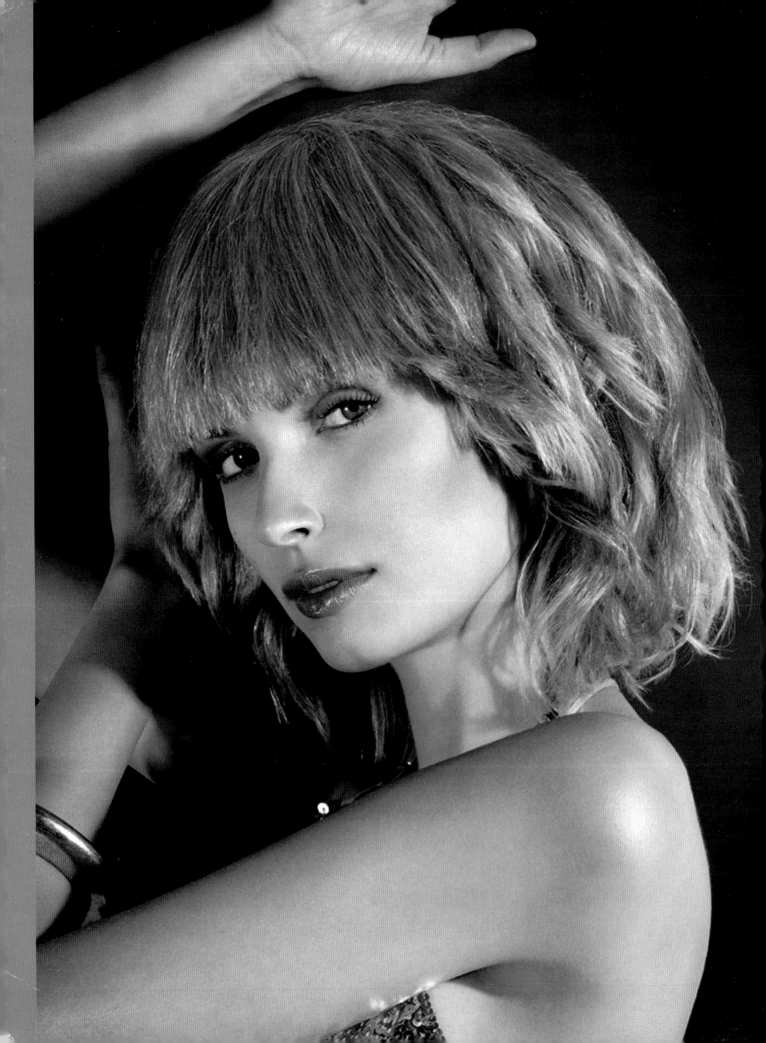

step by steps

" To be a great hairdresser you need to be both a strong artist and have excellent technique. Hairdressing is a very creative process and anyone in the industry will already have these essential skills. I travel the world with the Saks Art Team teaching Saks' signature techniques to encourage further development. It's important to take time out to look beyond the things you know, so travel, the arts, music, fashion and other elements of design are all reference points and allow us to develop our experiences. **"**

SAKS' ANDREW BARTON, BRITISH HAIRDRESSER OF THE YEAR

chapter 6

STEP BY STEPS

HAIRCUT   LEVEL 2 ONE-LENGTH LOOK

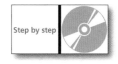

One-length look

Model   Emma
Stylist   Claire Morley, Contemporary

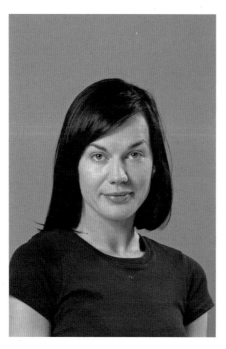

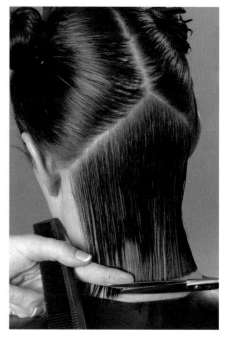

Step 1
Richesse de Diacolor 3 was used globally to give depth and shine to the hair. The hair was fine to medium in texture, and abundant, with no adverse hair growth patterns that would affect the haircut.

Step 2
A profile parting was made from the centre front hairline to the nape area. A diagonal subsection was taken from the centre of the head at the occipital bone. With the head slightly forward to reduce graduation, the first cut determined the length of the guideline and the finished look. Cutting continued to the top of the occipital bone.

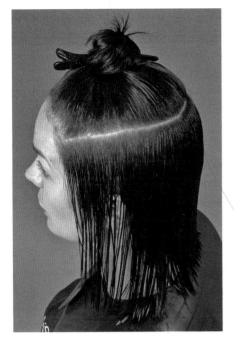

Step 3
A horse-shoe section was made from the front temple region over the crown area to incorporate the side sections.

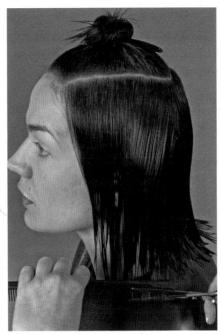

Step 4
The hair over the ear was cut without tension ensuring the overall length matches the lengths previously cut at the back.

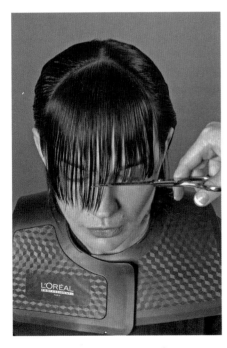

Step 5
The fringe was cut using a freehand cutting technique.

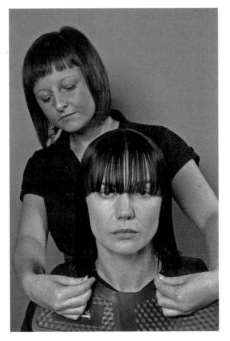

Step 6
The haircut was cross-checked to ensure that the hair length on both sides of the cut matched each other.

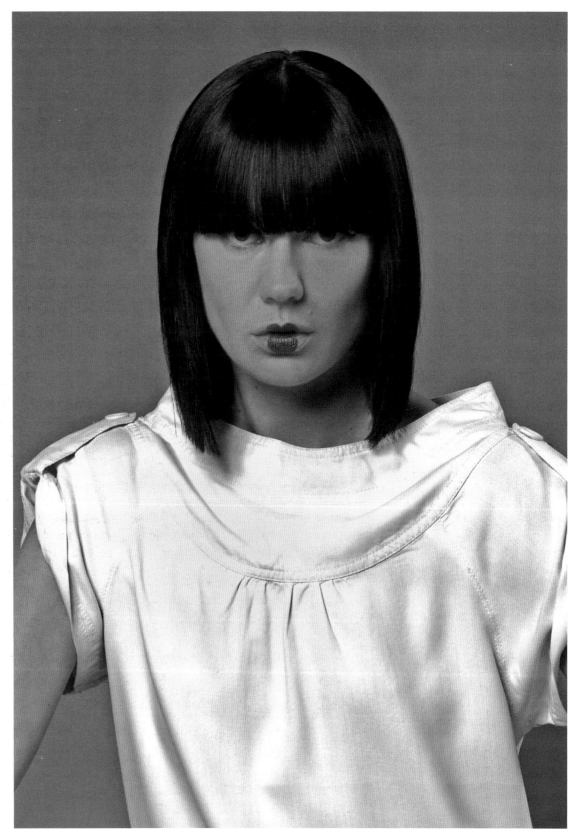

Step 7
The hair was finished to accentuate the precision cutting using irons with hot tecni.art style constructor – a heat-protective spray that nourishes the surface of the hair.

HAIRCUT   LEVEL 2 UNIFORM LAYER

Model   James
Stylist   Phil Gallagher, Headmasters

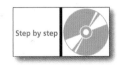

Uniform layer

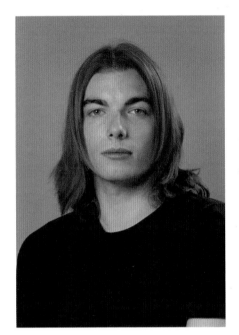

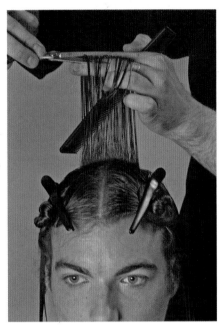

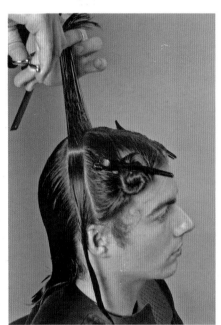

Step 1

The hair was fine with a slight wave. The hair was finer towards the front hairline with a cowlick from left to right. On the base colour of 7, Platinium Ammonia Free mixed with 20 volume hydrogen peroxide was woven into sections throughout the hair using Easi Meche Excel to create a soft sun-lightened look. Diacolor Gelée Dark Blond was used through the rest of the hair to create a natural even gloss.

Step 2

The hair was prepared for the haircut with tecni.art color show liss cream – a light, smoothing cream for coloured hair that tames frizz whilst enhancing colour and shine. The hair was sectioned from centre forehead to crown and then from ear to ear over the crown. The first 2 cm cutting section on the crown was taken from ear to ear. The hair was elevated to 90° from the head. The length cut determined the overall length of the haircut.

Step 3

The curve of the head was followed and a second section was taken down to the ear. This was repeated on the opposite side. The balance was checked by taking the hair just above the ears and pulling the hair up above the ears to ensure the hair is level on both sides.

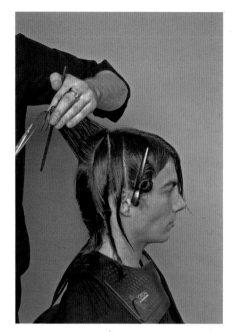

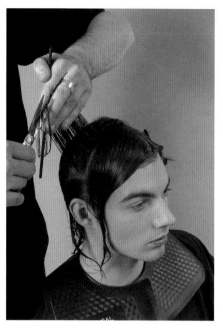

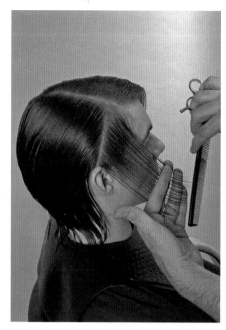

Step 4

A new section was taken from centre forehead to centre nape. This created a cross-panel guideline to work to. Using hair from the first section guideline, the hair was cut from crown to forehead and then crown to nape. Working from the centre back guideline, radial sections were taken from the crown to the nape, working forward towards the ear.

The work was cross-checked throughout the haircut. Remember, do not cut the hair during cross-checking without first going back to your original sections to check the lengths that the hair should be. You can correct any mistakes by cutting missed longer hair lengths.

The haircut was repeated on the opposite side.

Step 5

Parallel sections were taken from the crown using the crown profile line as the guideline. The haircut was continued by working forward towards the front hairline and continuing to cut the hair at 90° from the head.

The haircut was repeated on the opposite side.

Step 6

For the final finished cut, the baseline was checked to ensure that the cut was level. The front hairline was cut using short graduation. A section was taken from the recession area of the temple to the back of the ear. The hair at the base of the ear was cut softly, curving the hair towards the fringe area. The sideburns and nape hair were tidied with clippers.

The haircut was repeated on the opposite side.

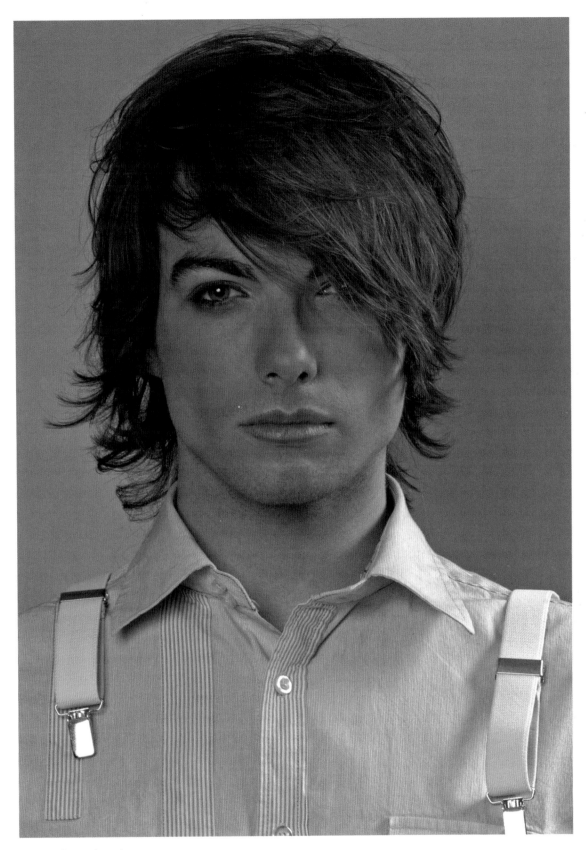

To finish and style
The hair was finished with L'Oréal Professionnel play ball beach crème – a soft, silky cream to texturise with a matt, beachy finish.

HAIRCUT   LEVEL 2 SHORT GRADUATION

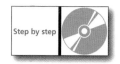

Model   Alicia
Stylist   Lyndsey Brockway, Level

Short graduation

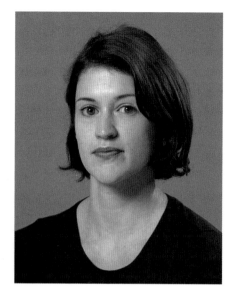

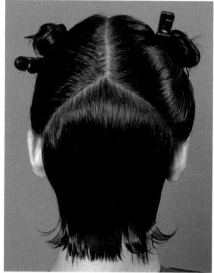

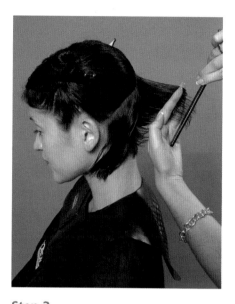

Step 1
The hair was abundant and the texture was fine. There were no adverse hair growth patterns. The hair was coloured using L'Oréal Professionnel Luocolor 4.15 and Easimeche back-to-back packets through the top sections alternating Luocolor 4.15 with Luocolor 5.6. This was to add depth, richness and texture within the panels.

Step 2
The hair was sectioned from centre forehead down to the centre occipital bone, then across the occipital bone from ear to ear.

Step 3
A vertical section was taken from the centre of the occipital bone down to the nape and the hair cut at 45° into the nape. The haircut was continued by taking vertical sections at 45° throughout the nape area. The hair was slightly overdirected towards the centre guideline to create length.

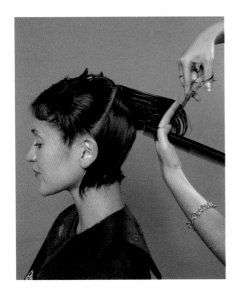

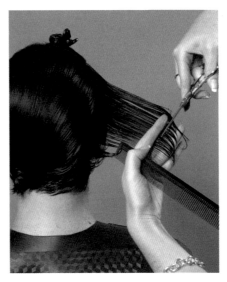

Step 4

Vertical sections at 45° were taken up to the crown using the previously cut hair as a guideline.

Step 5

Horizontal sections were taken from the temple to the ear. Using the previously cut hair as a guide, vertical sections were taken from the hair behind the ear. The hair was overextended into the guideline. Vertical sections were taken until there was no hair left to cut.

The haircut was repeated on the opposite side.

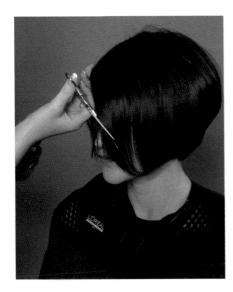

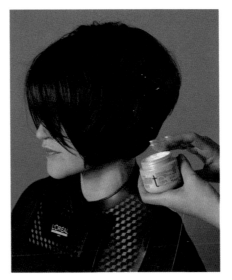

Step 6

The hair was dried into shape, following which, freehand cutting techniques were used to soften and personalise the fringe section.

Step 7

The hair was finished by defining and texturising the layers with tecni.art color show define wax – a cream wax especially designed for coloured hair.

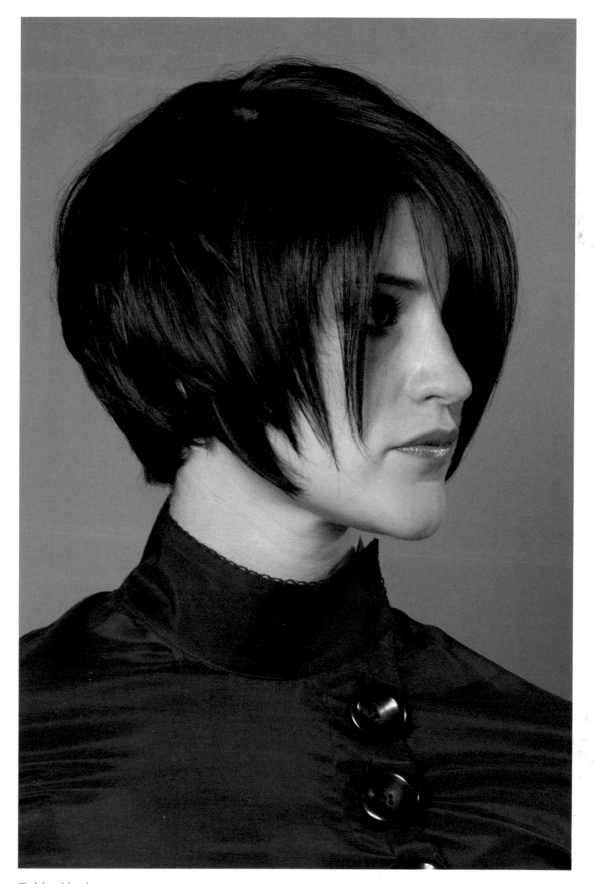

Finished look

HAIRCUT LEVEL 2 LONG GRADUATION

Model Mia
Stylist Andy Smith, John Carne

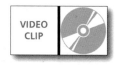

Long graduation

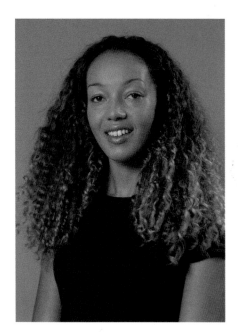

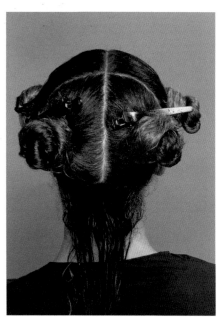

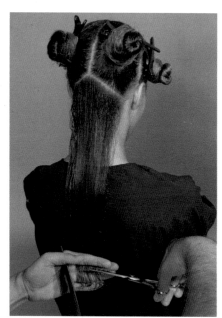

Step 1
Previous highlights were refreshed using Richesse de Diacolor Apricot Milkshake in 9.04. The hair was abundant, fine-textured African-type hair.

Step 2
To aid cutting, the hair was spritzed with série expert hydra repair – an ultra-light leave-in conditioning spray. To make the hair more manageable L'Oréal Professionnel tecni.art hairmix spiral splendour and sublime shine products were blended together and applied to the hair. The hair was sectioned from centre front to centre nape and then from ear to ear over the crown.

Step 3
A second section was taken 2.5 cm from the centre nape angling the section down to the ear. This helped to maintain the corners when cutting. The hair was club-cut to length making sure there was even tension on the hair. Sections were taken on both sides as the cut progressed to the crown.

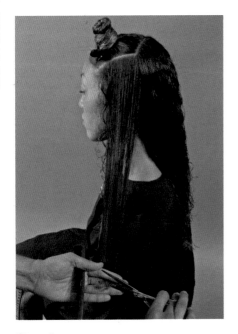

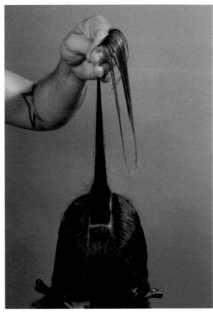

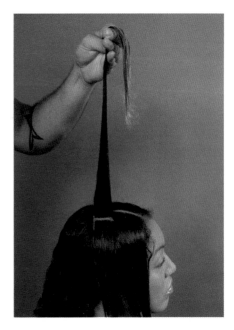

Step 4

The next cutting section was taken above the ear, slightly diagonal towards the front hairline to blend the sides with the back length. This created the external shape of the haircut. The cut continued up to the centre parting.

The haircut was repeated on the opposite side.

Step 5

The hair was re-sectioned from centre front to centre nape. With a 2.5 cm section, the hair was club-cut starting from the hairline and following the shape of the head working back to the crown. Then, from the crown to the nape, the hair was overdirected to create additional length towards the nape.

Step 6

The hair was re-sectioned from ear to ear over the crown. The section was as wide as the ear from front to back. Using the previously cut hair at the top of the crown as a cutting guide, the hair was overdirected to the last hair section above the ear towards the centre of the head, to create additional length.

L'Oréal Professionnel tecni.art hydro repair was used throughout the haircut making it easier for the hair to be combed through.

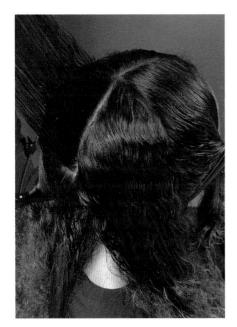

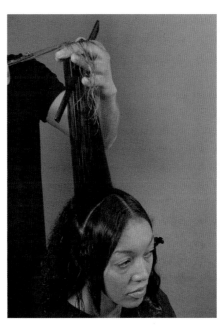

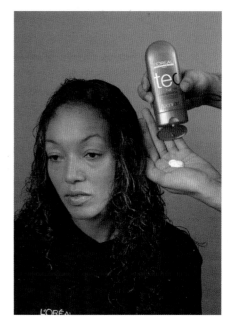

Step 7

The hair was re-sectioned from centre forehead to centre nape and from ear to ear over the crown. Then, using the centre back hair as a guide, the back two sections were taken using vertical sections to the ear to create internal layers.

Step 8

The front sections were taken vertically and overdirected back into the previously cut hair, then the cut was continued forward towards the front hairline.

The haircut was repeated on the opposite side.

Step 9

The hair was dried using L'Oréal Professionnel tecni.art and hairmix spiral splendour – a defining cream to nourish and control dry, thick, curly hair. The product was applied throughout the hair and the curls diffused.

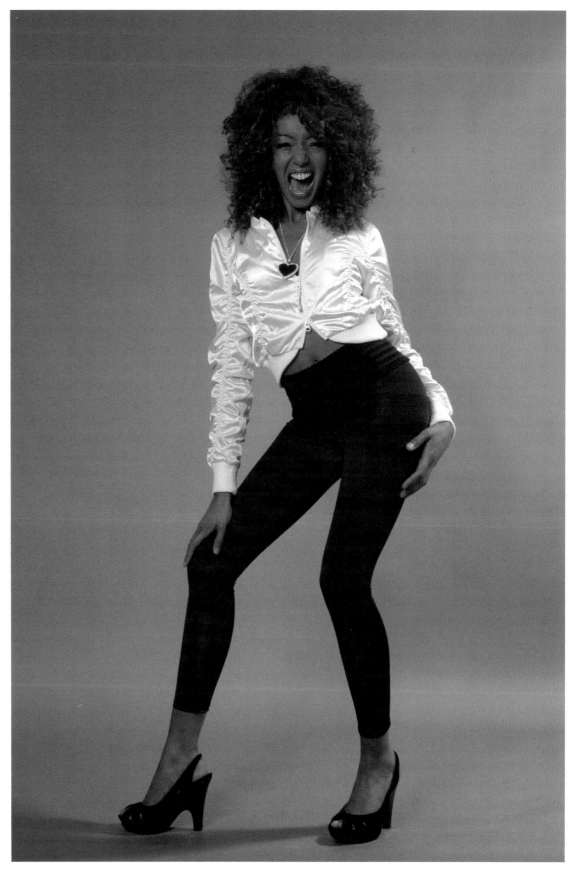

Finished look

HAIRCUT   LEVEL 3 CURRENT LOOK

Stylist   Toni & Guy

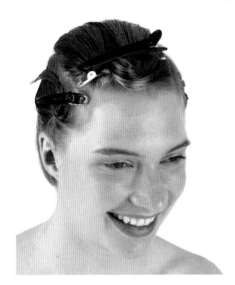

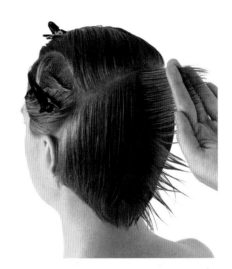

Step 1

The hair was fine. Prior to cutting the hair was coloured using an overall base colour to give depth. Sections of hair around the front and sides were woven out and coloured using majine and Easi Meche Excel and was used to create texture and definition to the finished haircut. The hair was sectioned from ear to ear over the crown and then from each temple back to the crown area.

Step 2

The first vertical cutting section was taken from the centre nape holding the hair at a 90° angle from the head. The hair was then point cut up to the crown.

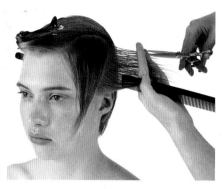

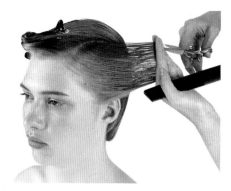

Step 3
The haircut was continued by using vertical sections, using the length from the first section as a guide, working towards the ear.

Step 4
Each section was overdirected back to the first guideline. This created length towards the front hairline.

The haircut was repeated on the opposite side.

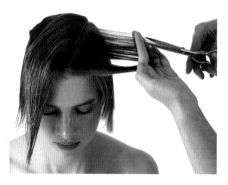

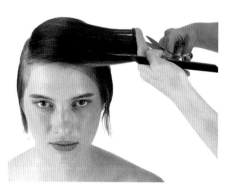

Step 5
The top section was cut. A horizontal section was taken, with the section held flat to the head to blend in to the previously cut hair.

Step 6
Horizontal sectioning was continued, overdirecting the hair back to the first horizontal guideline. This created additional length across the top front section. The haircut was personalised by point cutting into the top and sides to create additional texture and by creating a asymmetric fringe.

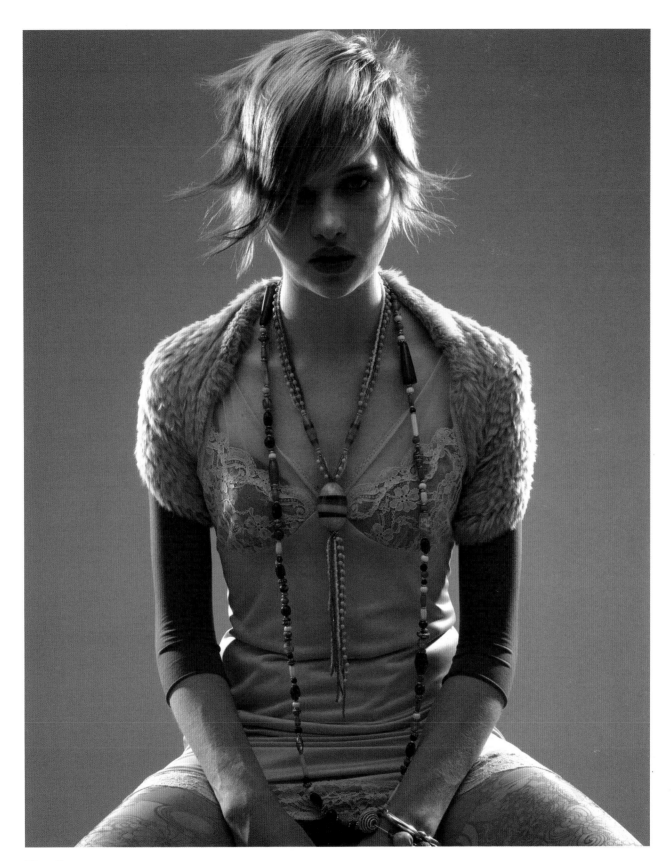

Step 7
The hair was finished with tecni.art play ball extrême honey worked through the ends to provide instant hold and a natural-looking shine.

HAIRCUT   LEVEL 3 GRADUATION

Stylist   Alan Edwards

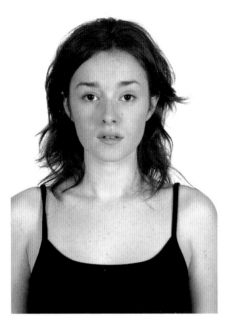

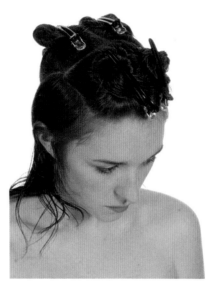

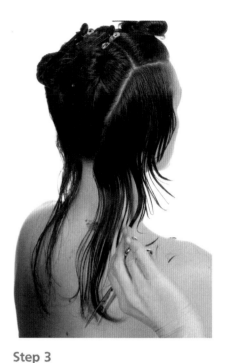

Step 1
The hair was medium in texture and abundance, slightly wavy with no adverse hair growth patterns.

Step 2
The hair was sectioned prior to cutting. The top sections were separated from the crown to nape area, leaving the hair from the sides of the front hairline to the nape of the neck free, ready for cutting.

Step 3
The exterior of the haircut was cut using a freehand technique to blend the short lengths at the front to the longer lengths at the back of the haircut. This was done by working section by section to the temple area and diagonally down into the nape. It was then repeated on the opposite side.

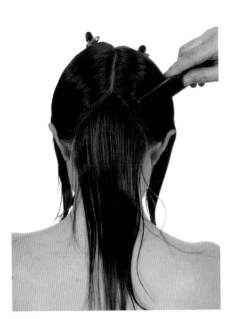

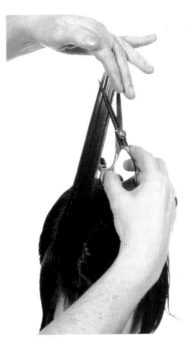

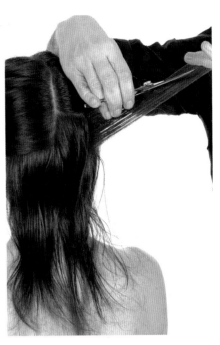

Step 4

The hair at the back was sectioned from the crown to the top of the occipital bone and then with 45° angles from the occipital bone to the nape area.

Step 5

To retain the length and create texture and movement in the hair, a vertical subsection was made. The hair was combed up and overdirected. The hair was cut using a slicing technique.

Step 6

The hair was held at a right angle to the scalp and, using the same slicing technique, it was cut from the top section to create texture within the interior of the haircut.

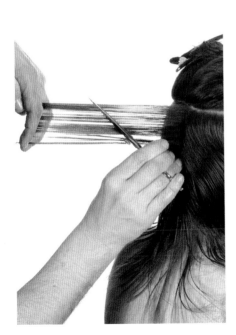

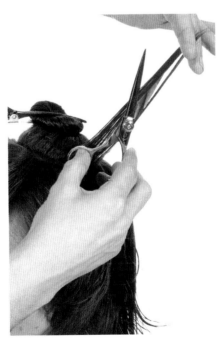

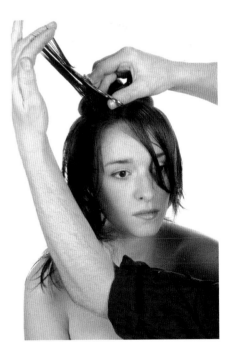

Step 7

To increase the texture further, the hair was sliced following a 45° angle on the underneath of the section.

Step 8

The same slicing technique was used throughout the haircut.

Step 9

The hair at the front hairline was sliced to create texture.

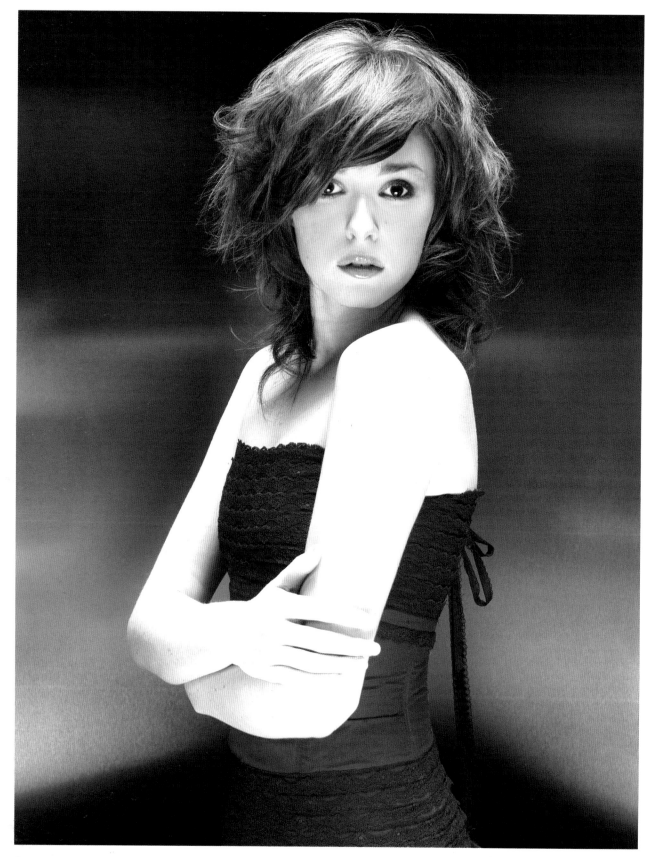

Step 10
The finished look was dressed with tecni.art fix arti-frizz to create volume and movement.

HAIRCUT   LEVEL 3 CLASSIC LOOK

Stylist   Toni & Guy

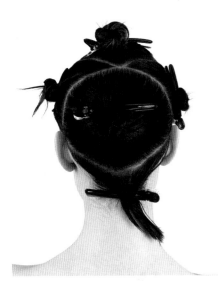

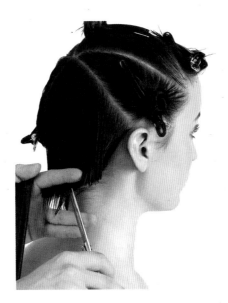

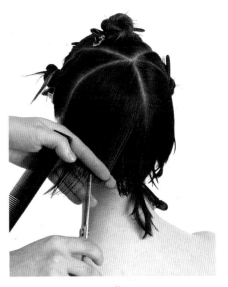

Step 1
The hair was prepared prior to cutting using a series of triangular-shaped sections. The hair at the nape was separated from the hair over the occipital bone and subdivided at the front and temporal regions.

Step 2
The nape was cut using a point-cutting technique to the desired length. The hair was held at an angle of 45° to create graduation.

Step 3
The hair at the occipital bone was blended into the nape hair, maintaining the graduated angle.

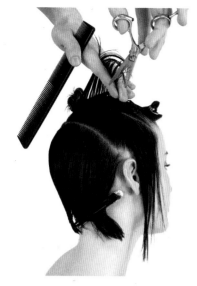

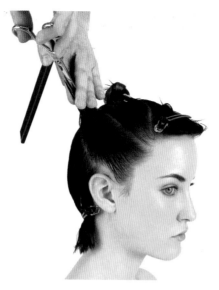

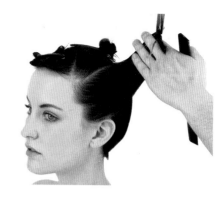

Step 4

The hair at the sides was held at a right angle from the scalp, with fingers held at an angle of 45° to create graduated layers within the haircut.

Step 5

The hair above the ears was directed towards the graduated layers and point cut to blend.

Step 6

The hair at the front hairline was overdirected to blend in the previously graduated layers.

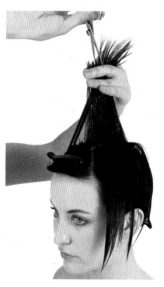

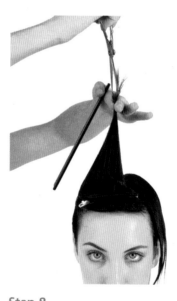

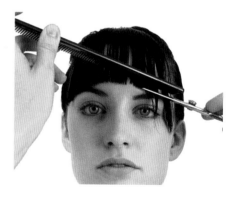

Step 7

The hair at the top of the head was held at right angles and point cut to create texture and movement at the ends of the hair.

Step 8

To ensure the hair length was maintained, the hair was overdirected and cut, at the same time ensuring the previously cut hair at the top was blended together.

Step 9

The fringe was club-cut to create a strong look and curved so that it was slightly shorter in the centre of the forehead.

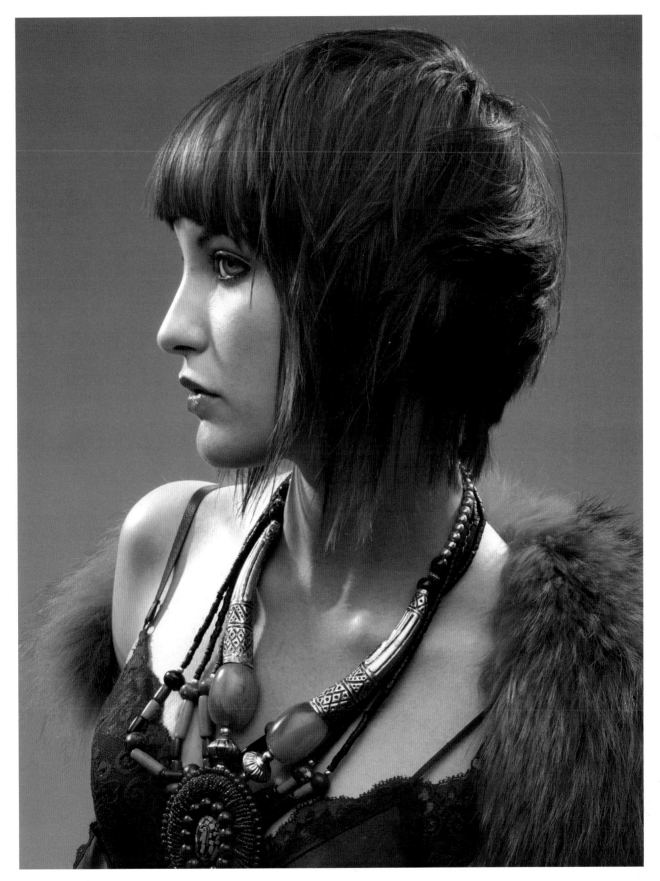

Finished look

HAIRCUT   LEVEL 3 CURRENT FASHION LOOK

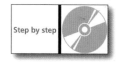

Step by step

Current fashion look

Model   Ben
Stylist   Herman Ho, Headmasters

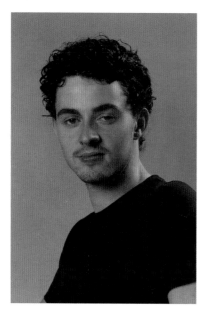

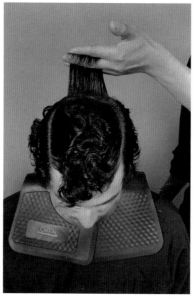

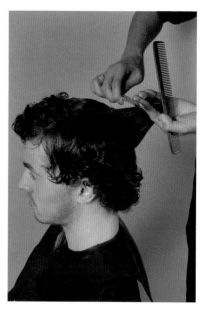

Step 1

The roots were natural base 6. The hair was gently cleansed using Efassor and warm water to remove the previous colour. L'Oréal Professionnel Luocolor 4.07 and 6.07 was used to add gloss and to create ultra-natural reflects. Then, Platinium mixed with 40 volume nutri-developer was painted on, using a freehand technique to break up and create texture within the style.

The hair was naturally curly, medium in texture and abundant. There were no adverse hair growth patterns.

Step 2

A horse-shoe section was taken from front recessional area through the crown area. The hair was held at a 90° angle and a point-cutting technique was used to reduce the length.

Step 3

The hair was sectioned from the crown to the occipital bone and a diverse graduation technique was used to reduce volume. This cutting technique was used to maintain the length at the occipital bone. Parallel sections were taken from the centre, working towards the ear on both sides, and maintaining the diverse graduation.

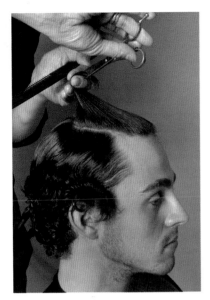

Step 4
The hair was overdirected from the front hairline and point cut using a guideline from the original cut length at the crown. This maintained the length for the fringe area.

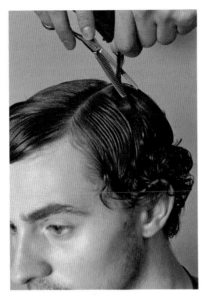

Step 5
A twist cutting technique was used through the front and sides to create texture and remove weight in the hair. Hair was twisted and cut using thinning scissors. The scissors were inserted at different levels two or three times into each twisted section.

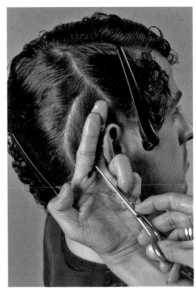

Step 6
Using a C section which followed the hairline growth pattern behind the ear, the hair was undercut. This reduced hair volume and produced a slimmer, masculine look.

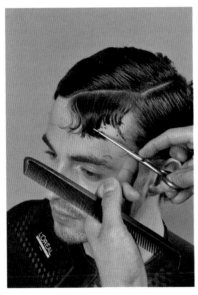

Step 7
The fringe was cut using a freehand technique to create asymmetry.

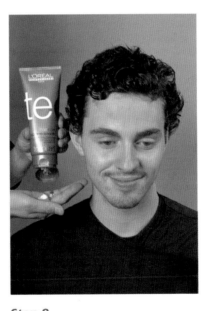

Step 8
The hair was dried and styled using tecni.art hairmix supreme smooth – a smoothing cream to condition and nourish thirsty, rebellious hair.

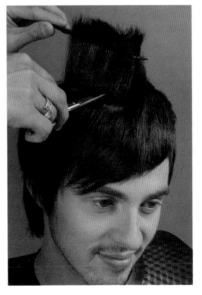

Step 9
Once the hair had been dried and straightened, a root slicing technique was used. Scissors were inserted into the root and sliced through from root to point separating the hair, creating texture and removing weight.

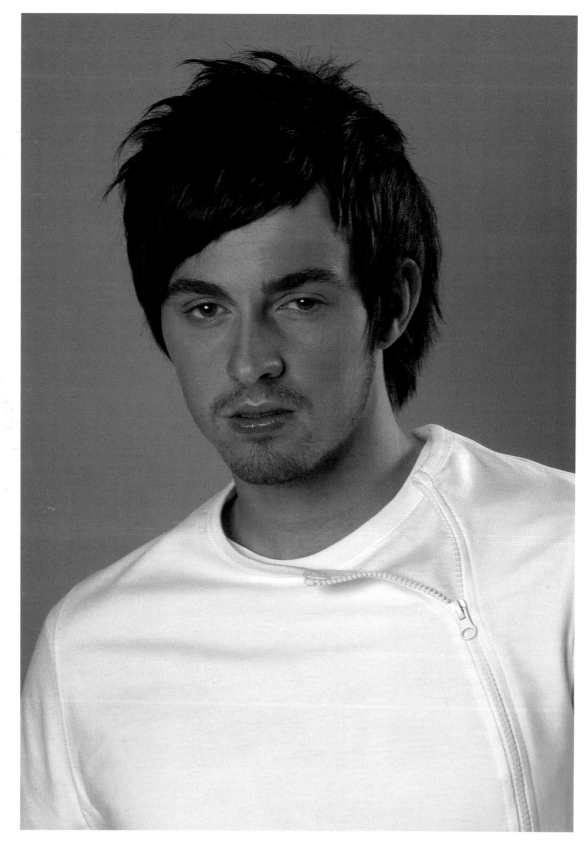

Step 10
The hair was finished with tecni.art hairmix sublime shine – a shine serum that tames and adds natural shine to very dry hair.

HAIRCUT   LEVEL 3 EMERGING FASHION LOOK

Model   Helen
Stylist   Tiziana Dimarcelli, Trevor Sorbie

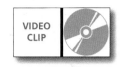

VIDEO CLIP

Emerging fashion look

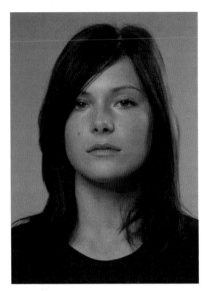

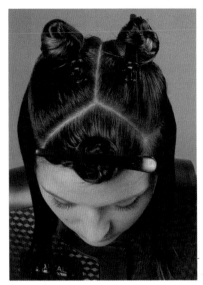

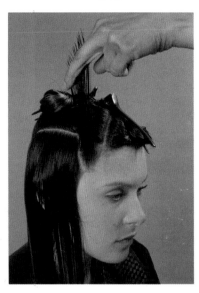

Step 1

The hair had been previously coloured and to add an intense gloss Diacolor Gelée Clear was used. The hair was medium in texture and abundant, with no adverse hair growth patterns.

Step 2

To prepare the hair for cutting tecni.art color show liss cream – a smoothing cream for coloured hair – was used.

The hair was sectioned from the centre front to the centre nape. A triangular section, approximately 5 cm deep, was taken from the centre front to the temple. A further curved section was taken from the temple to the occipital bone.

Step 3

At the temple, a diagonal section was taken and the hair was lifted by pointing the fingers towards the curved section in order to achieve the correct angle for the internal layers.

The hair was cut and the haircut continued, taking sections towards the centre nape.

The haircut was repeated on the opposite side.

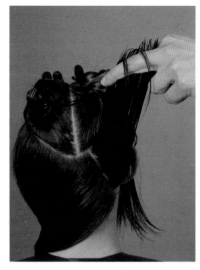

Step 4
The same angle was maintained through to the hair at the back and nape of the head.

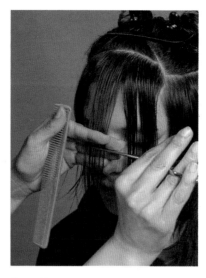

Step 5
The fringe was cut using horizontal sections and curving from the centre into the sides.

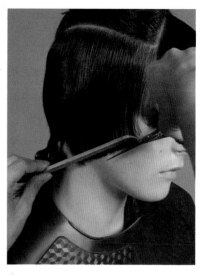

Step 6
The side section was joined into the fringe by using diagonal sections flat to the skin. Taking diagonal sections from the front hairline to the temple, the hair was directed forward onto the face. The haircut was continued by working back towards the ear.

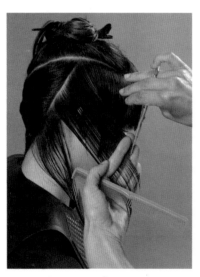

Step 7
From behind the ear to the nape, diagonal sections were taken and overdirected towards the front hairline, maintaining length at the centre back.

The haircut was repeated on the opposite side.

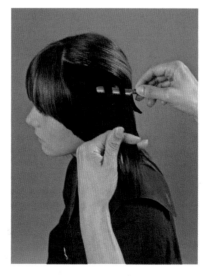

Step 8
On the disconnected top section a razor was woven through a section of hair and the underneath section of the hair was cut. This reduces weight. The haircut was continued by razor cutting the top section. The baseline was neatened with the scissors to give a clean sharp edge.

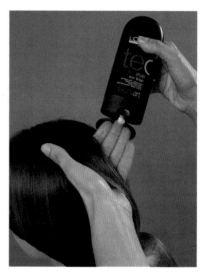

Step 9
To complete the finished look L'Oréal Professionnel tecni.art hot style iron finish was used – a heat-protective cream that provides the ultimate protection from the heat of irons, leaving the hair smooth and shiny.

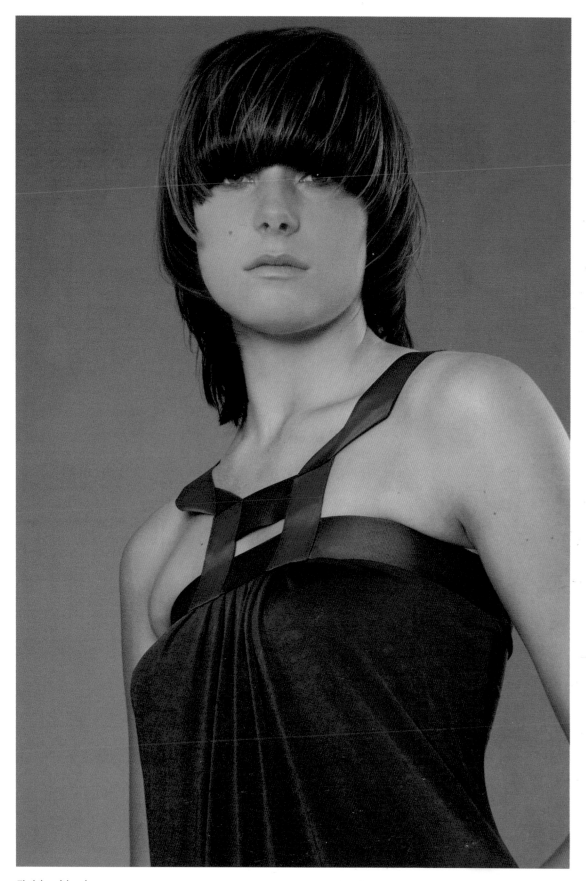

Finished look

HAIRCUT   LEVEL 3 AVANT-GARDE LOOK (FEMALE)

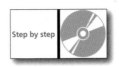

Avant-garde look
(female)

Model Tam
Stylist Carly Aplin, Cutting Room

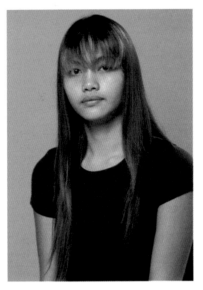

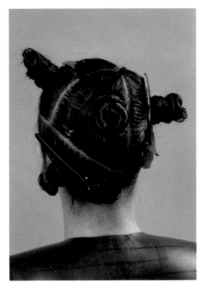

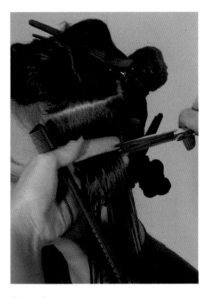

Step 1
The hair was abundant, medium-textured, Asian hair. There were no adverse hair growth patterns. The hair had a natural base colour of 3, which was coloured using Richesse de Diacolor 4 and 4.26 globally to create depth and give a glossy and rich reflect throughout the length and ends.

Step 2
The hair was sectioned from an off-centre parting through to the nape area. A second section was taken from the temple areas through to the nape to meet the first section. Approximately 2.5 cm of hair was left from the ear and below the parting. The section was disconnected from the internal haircut. A third section was taken from the crown down to meet the diagonal section 2.5 cm from the ear.

Step 3
The cut started on the opposite side from the parting. The first cutting section was taken from the temple to the ear.

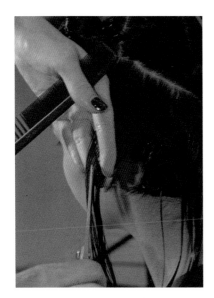

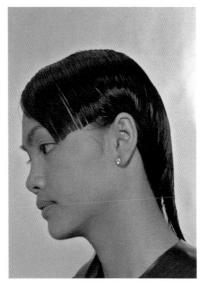

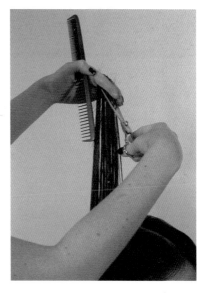

Step 4
The second cutting section was taken from the ear to the nape using the first cut section guideline. The hair was overdirected from the nape to maintain length and slight graduation.

Step 5
The sections were brought down until the parting was reached, using the previously cut hair as a guide.

Step 6
On the opposite side of the head a section was taken from the crown to the nape using the previously cut sections as a guide. The angle was overdirected and the scissors used to slice-cut the hair. Working towards the front hairline, the hair was continually overdirected to create additional length on each section.

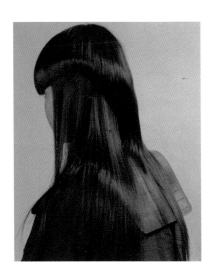

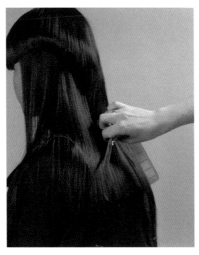

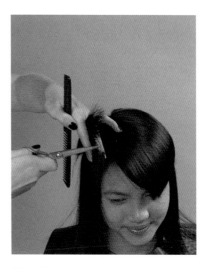

Step 7
The hair was dried using tecni.art liss control – a smoothing gel-cream that leaves the hair smooth and shiny.

Step 8
The dried hair was sliced to created disconnection to break up the length.

Step 9
The ends of the hair were shattered using texturising techniques and finished with Finish with tecni.art liss control+ – a smoothing serum that provides intense control and natural-looking shine.

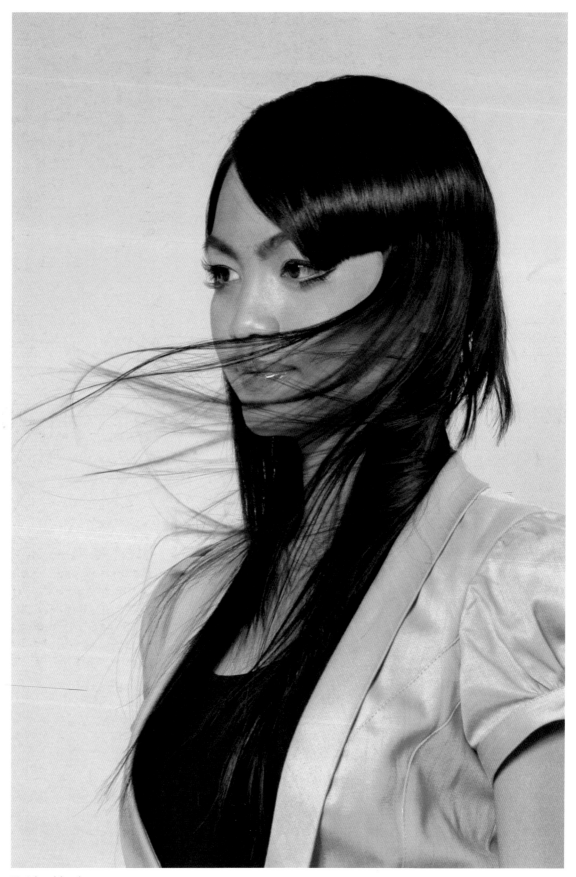

Finished look

HAIRCUT   LEVEL 3 AVANT-GARDE LOOK (MALE)

Model   Jon
Stylist   Jonny Engstrom, Guy Kremer

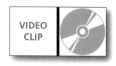

VIDEO CLIP

Avant-garde look (male)

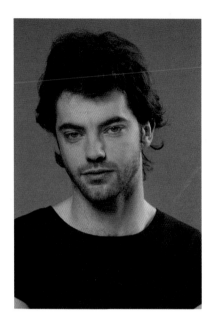

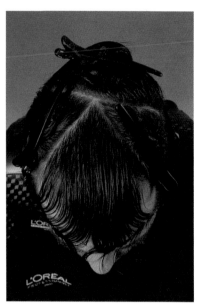

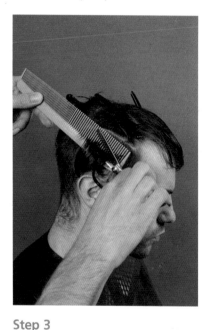

Step 1

To add gloss to the hair, Richesse de Diacolor 5.01 cool light brown was applied and left for 5 minutes to give an even depth throughout, keeping the reflect natural and cool which is ideal for men's colouring.

The hair was wavy, abundant and medium textured.

Step 2

Sections were made to identify the areas that were to be cut. The front triangular section was separated from the hair at the sides and back.

Step 3

The hair was cut using the scissor over comb technique on the sides and back of the head using 2.5 cm sections. Thinning scissors were used to create a soft finish to the very short hair that was undercut at the sides of the head. A jumbo comb was used to keep the hair separated during the haircut.

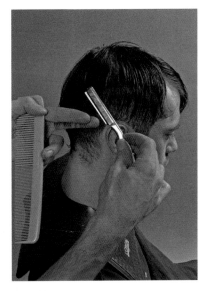

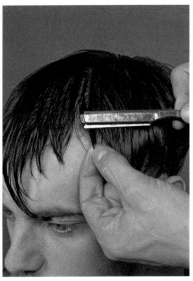

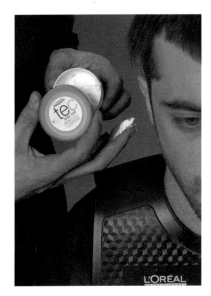

Step 4
The hair from the side sections was left to hang over the undercut and then cut on the edge with a razor to create texture and transparency on the ends of the hair. A panel over the occipital bone was left longer, cut into a point, creating added dimension to the look of the haircut.

Step 5
The recession areas were accentuated by cutting the hair back to the hairline with a razor in order to create a strong, pointed fringe. The outline of the fringe was personalised by picking up individual pieces of hair before cutting.

Step 6
A slicing technique was used on the top section to reduce length and weight. A choppy, layered effect was created by holding the hair at the tips to create space, and then slicing from under the fingers to the ends.

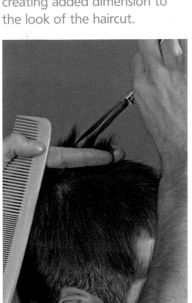

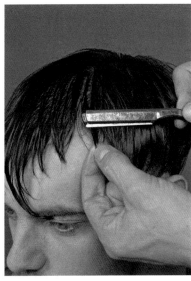

Step 7
After drying the hair, the top section was held at a right angle to the scalp and point cut to create texture.

Step 8
After the hair was dried it was finished with L'Oréal Professionnel tecni.art play ball density material – a texturising wax-paste that gives strong hold, definition and body to the hair with a matt finish.

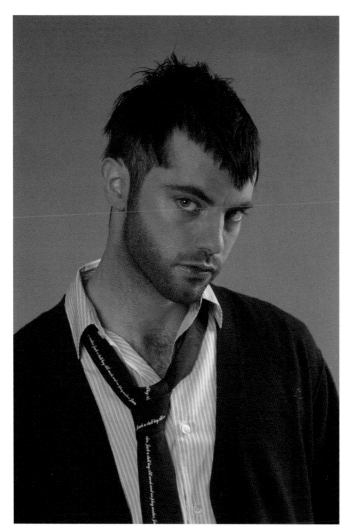

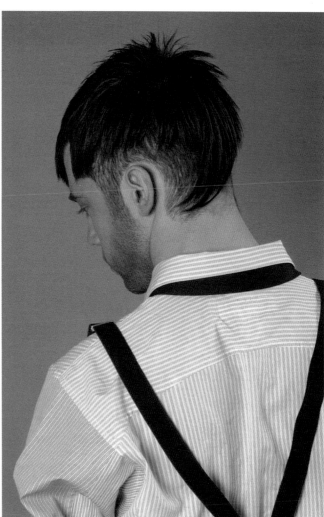

Step 9
Finished look.

HAIRCUT   LEVEL 3 PATTERNS IN HAIR

Stylist   Mucktaru Kargbo (MK), MK Hair Studio

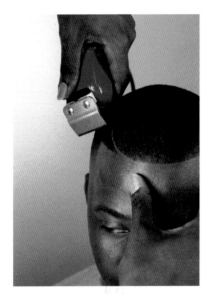

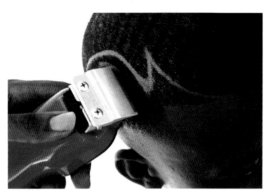

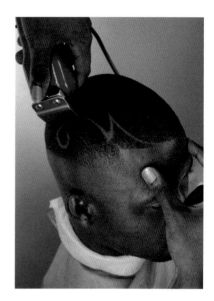

Step 1
The design parting was started by using the point of closed clipper blades which were set to zero.

Step 2
The pattern was worked over the parietal bone before the design was continued to the temporal area, the hair being combed to check that the lines were clean.

Step 3
The design was continued across the temporal bone with the curvature of the pattern being achieved by using the corner of the clippers.

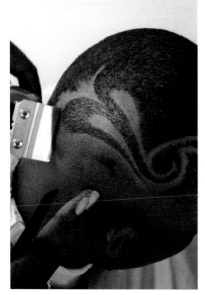

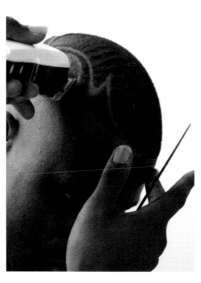

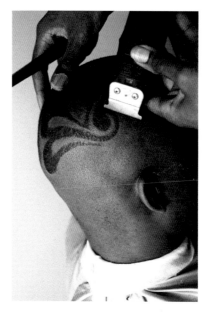

Step 4
The petal design was given definition and dimension by creating shading outside the original design line.

Step 5
Graduation was created underneath the design to form depth by reducing the level of hair.

Step 6
A T-blade clipper was used to create curvature and points; adjustable clippers were also used for graduated shading, allowing a two-dimensional effect to be seen.

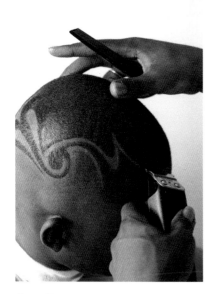

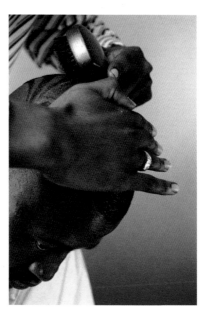

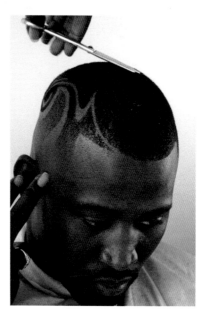

Step 7
The design was enhanced by ensuring that any minute hairs that may intrude on the precision cut lines were removed.

Step 8
The hair was brushed, following the hair growth patterns, and this was followed with the hand to remove static electricity, allowing the hair to lie flat.

Step 9
Scissors were used to remove stray hairs following the shape of the hairstyle and final design.

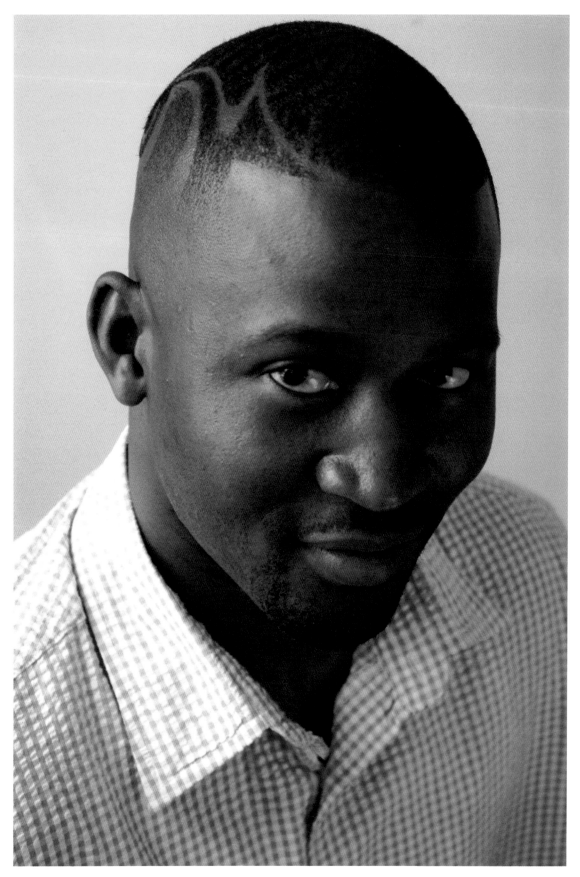

Finished look

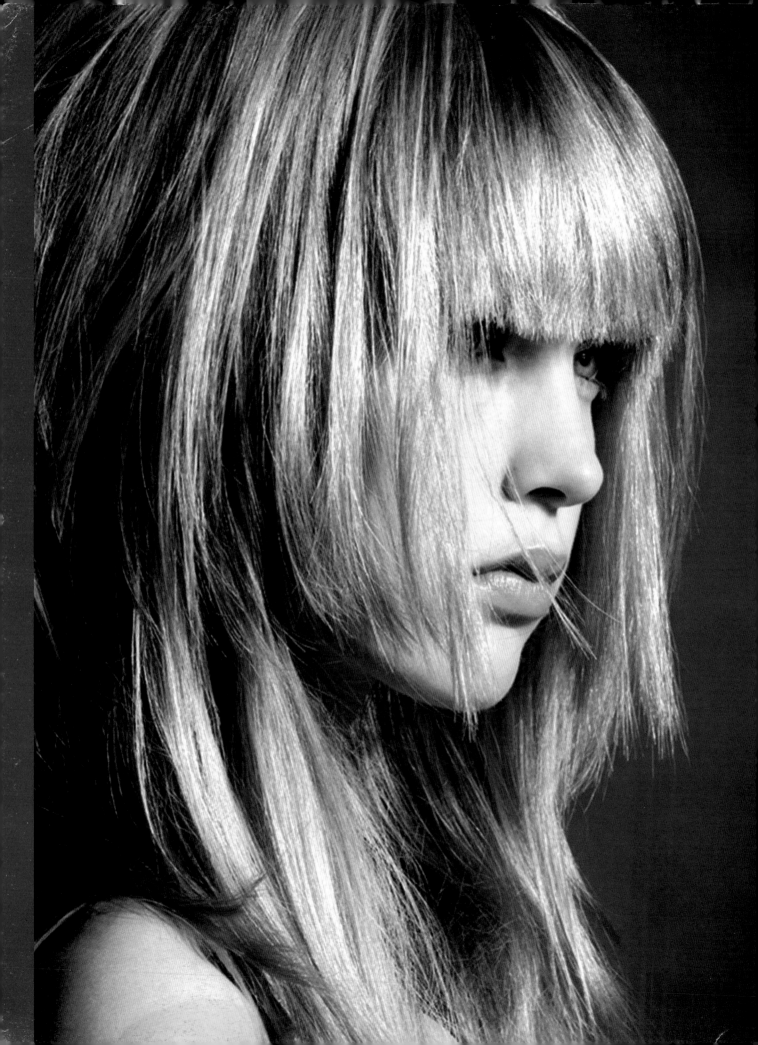

working safely in the salon

> **"** Hairdressing salons are a hive of activity and when busy can be a very exciting and even hectic environment to work in, therefore it is absolutely essential for the safety of your clients and your staff that you adhere to good and safe working practices. Only by having the correct systems in place is it possible to work feeling confident in the knowledge that risk has been kept to an absolute minimum. **"**

ANDREW COLLINGE

chapter 7

WORKING SAFELY IN THE SALON

Learning objectives

In this chapter you will learn about the knowledge you need to gain in order to work safely within the salon. You will learn about the health and safety regulations and legislation that will keep your clients, your colleagues and you safe from harm when in the salon. We will consider:

- **who the legislation is for**
- **why we need legislation**
- **who is responsible for safety in the salon**
- **client care and safety**
- **your personal appearance and conduct within the salon**
- **your posture**
- **sterilising tools and equipment**
- **how to identify hazards and risks**
- **regulations and legislation**
- **fire safety**

This chapter links to the following S/NVQ units

G1 Ensure your actions reduce risks to health and safety

INTRODUCTION

There you are watching the salon burn down. You have just managed to get out with your friends, workmates and clients. Someone left a cigarette burning and nobody bothered to check before putting it in the bin.

Can you image what it would be like if there were no health and safety salon policy or regulations to work to? The salon would be a dangerous place for you to work in and your client to visit. There would be no requirements to ensure that the salon environment was safe to work in, no need to ensure that you had the right amount of ventilation or heat. No need to make sure you had personal protective equipment to use when working with chemicals such as perm lotion and colours. Tools and equipment would not need to be cleaned and sterilised for every client and electrical equipment would not be checked to make sure it was safe to use.

Health and safety regulations are there to protect everyone – to make sure that you work in a clean and safe environment and that your client can expect you to provide a service using clean and hygienic tools and equipment which prevent bacteria, viruses, infections and infestations from spreading from client to client.

WORKING SAFELY IN THE SALON

As a hairdresser you might think that health and safety are not the sexiest words that spring to mind. When we think hairdressing we think about creativity, the fashion industry and glamour.

However, to become a good hairdresser we also have to follow health and safety regulations to ensure the safety of our clients, colleagues and ourselves. The subject of health and safety may seem uninteresting compared to carrying out haircutting or colouring services, but without understanding health and safety we will not be safe hairdressers or give good customer care.

It starts very simply with what the client sees when they enter the salon. Is the salon clean and tidy? Are the staff well presented and have they taken pride in their appearance? Throughout the client's visit they will be aware of what is happening around them and to them. It is important that you and your colleagues gain the trust and confidence of the client to ensure their visit is an enjoyable and safe one.

ACTIVITY

Walk around your salon and make a list of the objects, items or procedures that are making the salon look untidy, then identify if anything you have listed could cause an accident.

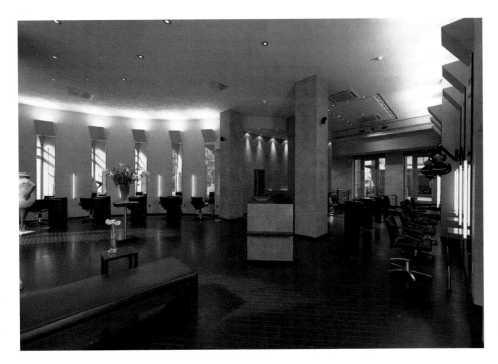

Salon portraying a professional image Saks

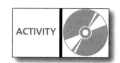

Spot the hazards

Spot the hazards in two salon images Habia

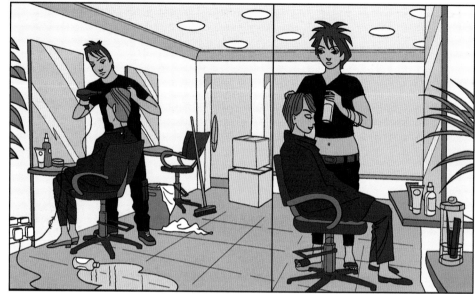

Who is health and safety legislation for?

Health and safety is for everyone in the salon: the employer, you the employee and your clients. There is a Health and Safety at Work Act (1974) that contains regulations to protect everyone within the workplace. It sets down the requirements that employers and employees must follow when they are working in a salon.

Why do we need legislation?

It does not matter what job or position you have in the salon, everyone needs to take responsibility for how they behave and the actions they take in the salon. You must be responsible for your actions, what they do and how that may affect colleagues and clients in the salon. Health and safety regulations and salon polices will ensure that everyone is aware of their own responsibilities for health and safety, and your job description should cover health and safety aspects such as:

- behaviour
- appearance
- use of drugs, alcohol and food
- working methods
- security.

Who is responsible for health and safety?

Everyone who works in the salon is responsible for health and safety. However, within your salon there may be designated person or several people responsible for different aspects of health and safety, such as:

- your employer or manager who has overall responsibility
- a person responsible for first aid
- a fire warden
- a person responsible for security.

It is important that you know to whom to go for help if an incident happens or to report a risk or hazard.

Client care

Health and safety is also a major part of client care. Communicating well with your client to find out what they want is all well and good, but if you then carry out the service in an unsafe way, your client will not have confidence in you or the salon and will probably not return. For example, if you fail to take care with the actions you use or the working environment, your client will not have confidence in you or the salon.

Clients want to be looked after and pampered during their visit. They will expect:

- to be given a clean gown to protect their clothing
- to be seated at a clean and tidy work station
- to be given a drink in a clean cup that is not chipped or stained
- to see that the towels used are freshly laundered
- combs, brushes and scissors to be sterilised before they are used
- you to work safely and responsibly while doing their hair.

Clients are paying for a total experience, not just the haircut. As a professional hairdresser it is your job to ensure your clients enjoy the experience and will look forward to their next visit. Part of the salon experience will be achieved by the way you present yourself to the client: by your appearance and your actions.

Personal appearance and conduct

Many salons will have an image that they want to portray to the world. They may want to attract a certain clientele – a certain age group or client spend. This image will often be reflected in what the salon owner expects you to wear in the salon and how you conduct yourself at work. This will usually be described in your job description. Your clients will also expect you to have a clean and tidy appearance and conduct yourself in a professional manner.

Personal appearance and conduct portrays not only the salon image but also your own personality. Even if you wear a salon uniform you need to take pride in your appearance. A clean and well-presented outfit will give the client confidence in you. If your clothes are dirty and soiled, it will mean the client receives a bad impression of you and the salon; it can also be disconcerting for your client and colleagues if you smell. Clothes that are restrictive and tight will not allow the air to circulate around the body and

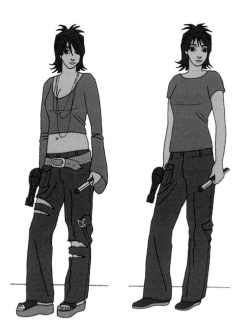

Stylists projecting an unprofessional and a professional image Habia

cause perspiration leading to body odour (BO). Your hair also reflects the salon image. It should be clean and well maintained at all times. Jewellery should not get in the way of work, and should not cause any discomfort to the client, by catching or pulling on them.

The way you conduct yourself at work will show your professionalism. Behaving sensibly and showing respect to your clients and colleagues are essential. Being aware of what is happening around you is important but you also need to concentrate on the work you are performing to ensure you do it safely.

Preparation is often the key to success. Before starting each new service it is important that you have prepared. You need to make sure that:

- your work station has been cleaned and prepared for your next client
- your tools and equipment have been cleaned and sterilised
- you have checked to see if your client has a record card
- you have the products you need available.

Many salons will have a work policy that will cover personal conduct, this will usually cover:

- time schedules for working
- reporting in when absent due to sickness or personal issues
- reporting incidents that may affect the salon or work colleagues
- the dress code
- salon smoking policy
- the mis-use of drugs and alcohol
- where and when eating and drinking can take place
- health and safety responsibility
- use of tools and equipment.

TIP	

Always read your salon's work policies. They will give you the information you need to work safely and responsibly.

Contact dermatitis

Contact dermatitis is a skin condition that can affect hairdressers. It is an itchy skin condition caused by an allergic reaction to certain materials. Rubber gloves or products such as shampoos that are in constant contact with the skin can cause irritation. In fact, one of the main causes of dermatitis for hairdressers is constantly having wet hands during the shampoo process. In some cases the condition can get so severe that the hairdresser may have to change their career. It is therefore important that after services such as shampooing hair or after cutting and styling a client's hair you wash and dry your hands and apply a good hand cream to protect them.

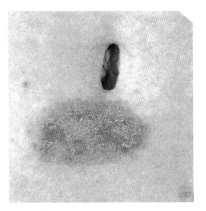

Contact dermatitis

Posture

Making sure your posture is correct is key to your long-term health and to the success of the cutting service you are carrying out. Bad posture will lead to body fatigue and possible long-term injury. Standing incorrectly will put pressure and strain on both muscles and ligaments. This happens when the upper part of the body is out of line with the lower parts. Bad posture will create pain and discomfort to you but also gives the client an impression of laziness and an uncaring attitude. Hairdressing is a tiring job; you are on your feet for the majority of the day; it is important that you are aware of the correct standing position to ensure your survival within the industry.

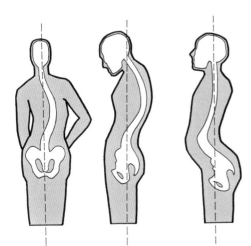

Postural faults Habia

Haircutting is about balance and accuracy. You must learn to have good posture to ensure that your stance is even and that you have good body balance as you work around the client during the haircut. Many hairdressers use a cutting stool to help maintain their body balance when cutting the lower sections of long hair or when working in the nape area on short hair.

Correct posture is achieved when your head, shoulders, upper body torso and abdomen, thighs and legs distribute your body's weight evenly over your feet, which should be facing forward and slightly apart. If you move position and lower one of your hips it will change the balance of your body and put more weight on that leg and foot. It will cause the spine to curve and put strain on the lower part of your back.

Sterilising tools and equipment

Sterilisation is the complete eradication of living organisms.

You must never use dirty tools and equipment. They must be cleaned and sterilised before they are used on your clients. As part of the consultation you will be identifying the tools and equipment you will need for the haircut. There will include combs, scissors and possibly a razor or clippers, and it is up to you to ensure that they are ready to use and fit for purpose.

Different tools and equipment are sterilised or disinfected in different ways. There are three main methods of sterilising tools. These are:

- heat
- radiation
- chemicals.

Within the hairdressing salon this will equate to:

- heat = the use of an autoclave
- radiation = the use of an ultraviolet light box
- chemicals = the use of barbicide.

Heat

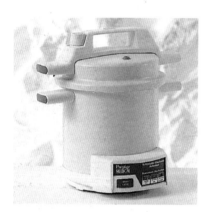

Autoclave

Autoclaves are the most reliable method of sterilising but not often used within the salon. They are used for sterilising metal tools such as your scissors. They work by building up steam pressure, creating heat that destroys all living bacteria.

Radiation

The ultraviolet (UV) light box is often used as a method of sterilising cutting tools. The tools must be washed and dried before they are placed in the box. The ultraviolet light will prevent bacteria growth on the tools but complete sterilisation is not guaranteed as tools will only be sterilised on the areas were the UV rays reach, so the tools must be turned over to ensure they have been exposed to the light on all sides. Because this method of sterilising is time-consuming and sterilisation cannot be guaranteed it is often better to use the UV light box as a hygienic method of storing tools that have already been sterilised by another method, rather than storing them in your tool bag.

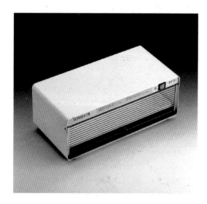

Ultraviolet light box

Chemicals

The use of chemicals is the most common method in the salon for disinfecting cutting tools. In hairdressing we tend to use a chemical called *barbicide*. It is a clear, blue, low-level disinfectant which does not sterilise tools but reduces the probability of infection. Barbicide must be changed daily and all the tools must be totally submerged in the solution and left in it for the time recommended by the manufacturer.

How to use barbicide solution:

- Tools such as combs and scissors must be cleaned with soap or detergent and a brush under running water prior to being placed in the barbicide.
- Barbicide must be made fresh daily. It will lose strength the more it is used and the longer it is kept.
- Tools must be fully immersed in the barbicide solution.
- Tools must remain in the solution for the required contact time. This is usually ten minutes, but follow the manufacturer's instructions.
- Rinse the tools under running water, or let them air dry depending on manufacturer's instructions.
- Place the clean, disinfected tools in a clean container to prevent contamination from other dirty items or the environment. **Do not** store clean and dirty tools together.

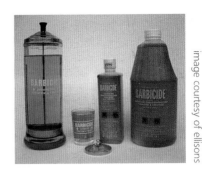

image courtesy of ellisons

Barbicide jar

Hazards and risks

It is your duty to be aware of potential hazards and risks in the salon. You need to be alert to spot a hazard that may become a risk to prevent an accident happening. If you can deal with a hazard make sure you do it quickly and safely; however, if you spot a hazard or risk that you cannot deal with make sure you inform the person responsible for health and safety.

- A *hazard* is something with the potential to cause harm.
- A *risk* is the likelihood of (someone being harmed by the hazard) the hazard's potential being realised.

For example:

- If a tap was leaking it could be classed as a hazard. If that tap was at the backwash area and the leak was creating a pool of water were colleagues stand to wash hair this would then be a risk, as the likelihood is that someone will slip and hurt themselves.
- If hair cuttings have been swept to the side wall of the salon this could be classed as a hazard. However, if the hair cuttings have been left on the floor around a work station then this would be a risk as the likelihood is that someone will slip and hurt themselves.

Hazard symbols

ACTIVITY

Draw a salon structure, similar to a family tree. Start at the top with the salon owner or manager and work down. Identify each person in the salon, what job they do and whether they have specific duties/responsibilities such as first aider.

ACTIVITY

Carry out a risk assessment in your salon. On the risk assessment form, list the hazards you have identified, the people who are at risk from the hazard and the existing procedures in place or additional procedures that are required.

ACTIVITY

Draw a diagram of your salon. Over a period of one to two weeks mark on the diagram if you identified a hazard and how you dealt with it.

IT'S A FACT

The Health and Safety Executive is responsible for health and safety in the workplace.

Risk assessment

The employer must carry out a risk assessment. It must cover all the activities that take place in the salon and the substances that are used within the salon.

A risk assessment is nothing more than a review of what in the salon could cause harm to staff and clients, so that your employer can weigh up whether enough precautions have been taken to prevent harm or if additional precautions needs to be put in place. The whole aim is to make sure that no one in the salon gets hurt or becomes ill.

The main thing your employer needs to decide is whether a hazard is significant and if sufficient procedures have been put in place to deal with the hazard satisfactorily.

How to assess the risks in your salon:

- Look for the hazards.
- Decide who could be harmed and how.
- Evaluate the risks and decide whether the existing precautions are all right or whether you need to do more.
- Record your findings.
- Review your risk assessment records and revise them when necessary, for example, if there are changes to the salon equipment or products.

HEALTH AND SAFETY REGULATIONS AND LEGISLATION

Your employer has a duty to protect you and keep you informed about health and safety; however, you have a responsibility to look after yourself and to work in a healthy and safe manner.

The Health and Safety Executive (HSE) is the organisation appointed by the government to support employers but also enforce health and safety laws, checking that employers are following all guidelines.

The Health and Safety at Work Act (1974)

The Health and Safety at Work Act (1974) is the main piece legislation from which most other legislation proceeds. The Act places a general duty of care on the employer to ensure, so far as is reasonably practical, the health, safety and welfare at work for all their employees. However, everyone at work has a responsibility to comply with the Act, including employees and trainees.

Employer's responsibility:

- Provide and maintain safety equipment and safe systems of work.
- Ensure products and equipment are properly stored, handled and used.
- Provide information, training and supervision and ensure all staff are aware of and use manufacturers' instructions.
- Provide a safe place of work.

- Provide a safe working environment.
- Provide a written safety policy/risk assessment.
- Look after the health and safety of clients.

Employee's responsibility:

- Take care of your own health and safety.
- Take care of the health and safety of colleagues and clients.
- Cooperate with your employer.
- Correctly use tools, equipment and products.
- Not to interfere with or misuse anything provided for health and safety purposes.

Health and Safety (First Aid) Regulations (1981)

People at work can have accidents or become ill. It is important that if you become ill or have an accident that you receive immediate attention. The Health and Safety (First Aid) Regulations requires your employer to provide adequate and appropriate equipment, facilities and personnel in the salon.

The minimum requirement is the provision of:

- a suitably stocked first aid box
- an appointed person to be responsible for first aid arrangements (but who will only attempt to give first aid if they have been trained).

There is no standard list of items that should be put in the first aid box. It depends on the working environment and what your employer has assessed the needs as being. However, a suggested minimum stock of first aid items will include:

- a leaflet giving general guidance on first aid e.g. the HSE leaflet on first aid at work;
- 20 individually wrapped sterile adhesive dressings (assorted sizes);
- 2 sterile eye pads;
- 4 individual wrapped (sterile) triangle bandages;
- 6 safety pins;
- 6 medium-sized individually wrapped sterile unmedicated wound dressings;
- a pair of disposable gloves.

Record keeping

It is a legal requirement for the employer or the designated responsible person to record in a book any incidents involving accidents, injuries and illness which have taken place and been attended to.

The following information should be included:

- date, time and place of incident;
- name and job of injured or ill person;
- details of the illness or injury and any first aid given;

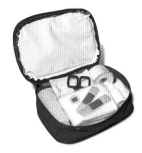

A first aid kit

TIP

How to deal with severe bleeding:

- Protect yourself from direct contact from the other person's blood.
- Apply direct pressure to the wound.
- Raise and support the injured part (if possible).
- Apply a dressing and bandage firmly in place.

TIP

How to deal with an eye injury:

- If there is something in the eye, wash out the eye using an eye bath with clean water or sterile fluid to remove loose items such as hair cuttings.
- If a chemical such as perm solution has entered the eye wash it out for at least 10 minutes, place a pad over the eye and send the client to the hospital.
- Do not attempt to remove anything that is embedded in the eye – seek medical attention.

- what happened to the casualty immediately afterwards, for example did they stay at work or go home or to the hospital;
- name and signature of the person dealing with the incident.

The records can help identify accident trends and improvement assessments to health and safety risks.

The Workplace (Health, Safety and Welfare) Regulations (1992)

This regulation provides your employer with a code of practice to maintain a safe, secure working environment. The requirements of the regulations cover:

- maintenance of the workplace and equipment e.g. that systems are in place to ensure the working environment is in efficient order and equipment is maintained and in good working order;
- ventilation e.g. that effective and suitable provision is made to ensure the salon is ventilated by a sufficient quantity of fresh or purified air;
- temperature in indoor workplaces e.g. that the temperature of the salon is reasonable;
- lighting e.g. that the salon has suitable and sufficient lighting;
- cleanliness and waste materials e.g. that the surfaces and floor etc. inside the salon are capable of being kept sufficiently clean;
- work stations and seating e.g. that they are suitable for the work to be carried out;
- conditions of floors and traffic routes e.g. that the floor is suitable for the working environment, easy to clean, not slippery and kept free from obstructions;
- windows and translucent doors and walls e.g. that they are appropriately marked or contain features that make the object noticeable.

The Manual Handling Operations Regulations (1992)

This regulation is about safe handling and manual lifting and the procedures employers need to put in place to ensure the safety of any staff moving heavy items. In the salon this could relate to product deliveries from manufacturers or moving chairs during cleaning activities. The regulations require the employer to carry out a risk assessment of activities that require manual lifting.

This should cover:

- the risk of injury
- the type of activity required such as strenuous pushing or long carrying distance
- if the loads will be heavy or difficult to handle
- the working environment such as slippery floors or variations in levels
- the staff's ability to handle and lift the objects
- training needs for staff.

Safe lifting practices

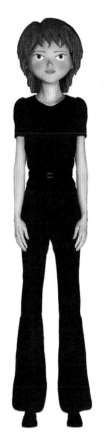

Stand with your feet apart

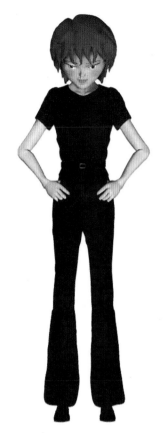

Your weight should be evenly spread over both feet

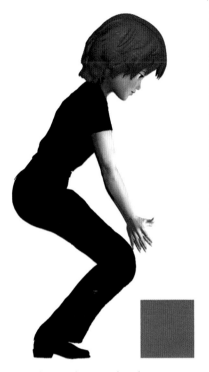

Bend your knees slowly keeping your back straight

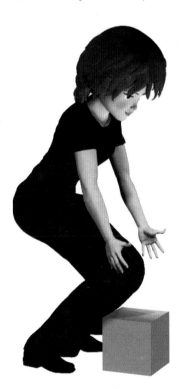

Stand with your feet apart

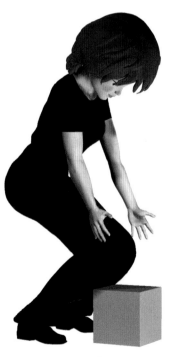

Tuck your chin in towards your chest

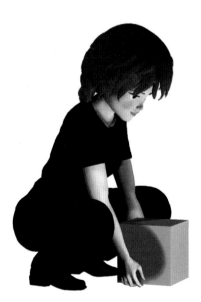

Get a good grip on the base of the box

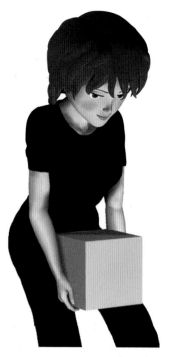

Bring the box to your waist height keeping the lift as smooth as possible

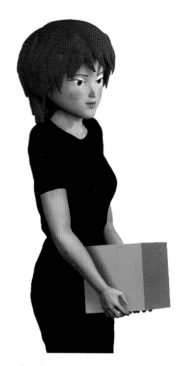

Keep the box close to your body

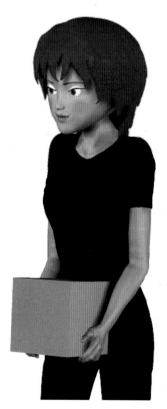

Proceed carefully making sure that you can see where you are going

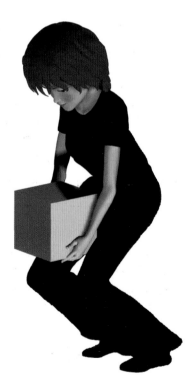

Lower the box, reversing the lifting procedure

The Provision and Use of Work Equipment at Work Regulations (PUWER) (1998)

This regulation is for employers and requires that equipment provided and used at work is:

- suitable for its intended use
- safe to use, maintained and if required inspected to ensure it is safe for use
- only used by staff that have received adequate information, instruction and training.

Personal Protective Equipment (PPE) at Work Regulations (1992)

This regulation requires the employer to provide personal protective equipment (PPE) that is to be used in the salon by staff when ever there is a risk to health and safety such as when using chemicals during perming and colouring services. The regulations require that PPE is:

- properly assessed before used to ensure it is suitable
- maintained and stored properly
- provided with instructions on how to use it safely
- used correctly by staff.

Control of Substances Hazardous to Health (COSHH) Regulations (1999)

Using chemicals such as perms, colours, hydrogen peroxide and bleach can put your health at risk, so the law requires your employer to control the use and exposure to hazardous substances to prevent ill health. COSHH regulations relate to the safe handling, storage and use of products. If they are not used correctly they may:

- cause skin irritation or dermatitis as a result of skin contact
- cause asthma if you develop an allergy to the substance
- cause you to lose consciousness as a result of fumes.

To make sure you are safe your employer will carry out a risk assessment of the products used in the salon and you as the employee must follow the salon's policy and manufacturers' instructions on how to use, handle and dispose of the products safely.

Electricity at Work Regulations (1989)

Electrical equipment is used all the time in the salon. One of the most common tools in haircutting is electric clippers. It is essential that clippers

Using electrical equipment

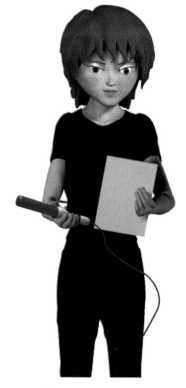

Know how to use it

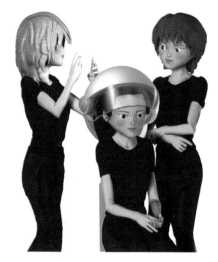

Be trained in its use

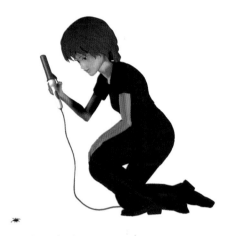

Use it only for the purpose intended

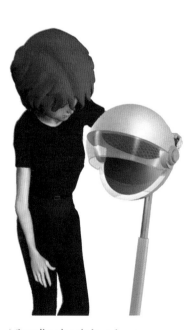

Visually check it prior to use

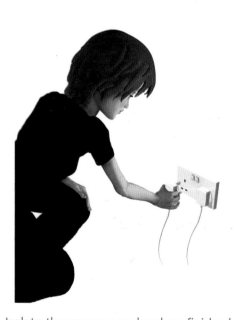

Isolate the power supply when finished

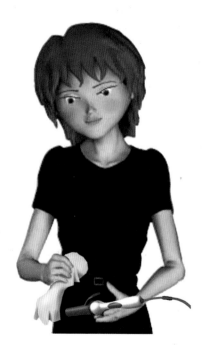

Clean equipment after each use

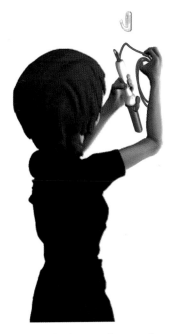

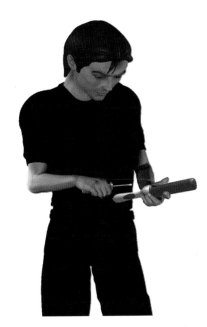

Store safely, in an allocated area

Have it tested regularly by a qualified electrician

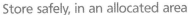

and all other electrical equipment is checked to make sure they are in good working order. The Electricity at Work Regulations requires your employer to maintain electrical equipment and have it checked by a qualified electrician every year. These checks must be recorded and the records made available for inspection. Your employer must provide suitable training to ensure that staff know how to use to equipment safely.

Your responsibility is to ensure that you visually check the electrical equipment before you use it; for example: are the wires secure at the plug?

If the equipment becomes faulty during use, for example, overheating or cutting out, you need to report the fault to a responsible person and label it as faulty before putting it out of use.

Reporting of Injuries, Diseases and Dangerous Occurrences Regulations (RIDDOR) (1995)

This regulation requires the employer to inform the Health and Safety Executive of work-related accidents, diseases and dangerous occurrences including:

- death
- fracture of the arm or leg (not the hand or wrist or ankle or foot) spine, pelvis or skull
- amputation of the hand or foot

- serious eye injury (this also includes chemical accidents)
- electrical shock requiring medical attention or loss of consciousness
- any injury requiring hospital admission as an in-patient for more than 24 hours
- an accident resulting in more than three days off work
- work-related diseases.

FIRE SAFETY

Fire safety is crucial for all salons. It is important that all staff in the salon are aware of the salon's safety procedures when it comes to:

- dealing with a fire
- evacuation procedures.

All staff should be know the type of fire extinguishers in the salon and were they are kept.

There are three things that must be present at the same time in order to create a fire:

- FUEL
- OXYGEN
- HEAT.

The combination of these three things is often referred to as a 'fire triangle'. Without one of these three components there will be no fire or the fire will be extinguished.

There are three methods of extinguishing a fire:

- cooling – the fire is extinguished by reducing the temperature;
- starving – the fire is extinguished by limiting or removing the fuel;
- smothering – the fire is extinguished by limiting or excluding oxygen.

There are three ways in which a fire spreads:

- conduction – this is when heat is passed through a material such as wood and metal;
- convection – this happens when a liquid or gas is heated;
- radiation – this is when heat is transmitted without contact.

There are five categories that classify fires:

- Class A – solid, organic materials
- Class B – liquids
- Class C – gases
- Class D – metals
- Class F – liquefiable solids such as fats and cooking oils.

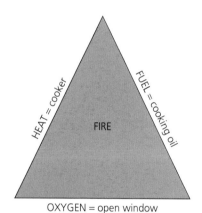

Fire triangle

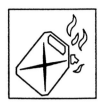
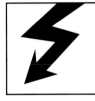

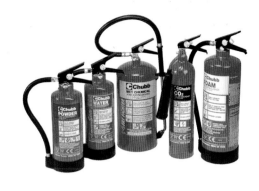

Fire extinguisher symbols

Fire extinguishers

Images courtesy of Chubb Fire Ltd.

Types of fire extinguishers.

Type of extinguishers	Classification of fire	Dangers
Water	A	Do not use on electrical fires or on burning liquids
Dry powder	A, B, C and electrical	Causes powder dust when used which could impair visibility
Wet chemical	A and F	Do not use on a fire that includes live electrical equipment
CO_2 (carbon dioxide)	B and electrical	Do not use in confined spaces and be aware of possibility that the fire may reignite particularly if fire is very hot
AFFF (aqueous film foaming foam)	A and B	Not generally used on fires with electrical apparatus

Only staff who have had training should use a fire extinguisher. Remember the most important thing to do is think safety first – raise the alarm if you see a fire and then quickly follow the salon's policy for evacuating the salon.

Assessment of knowledge and understanding

Test yourself on the content of this chapter by answering these questions.

Assessment activity level A

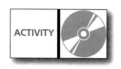

Working safely in
the salon

Link the legislation on the left with the reason for the legislation on the
right. You may use different coloured markers to show your connections.

Workplace (Health, Safety and Welfare) Regulations 1992	Wearing gloves and apron
Health and Safety at work Act 1974	Ensuring adequate ventilation
Provision and Use of Work Equipment Regulations 1992	Disposal of perm and colour products
Personal Protective Equipment at Work Regulations 1992	Main legislation in which nearly all other regulations are made
Control of Substances Hazardous to Health (COSHH) Regulations 2002	Ensuring the correct and safe operation of salon equipment

The answers to this activity can be found at the end of the book.

Activity level B

1 What is the main legislation under which nearly all other
   regulations are made?

2 What is meant by the term 'hazard'?

3 What is meant by the term 'risk'?

4 What is the name of the body appointed to support and enforce
   health and safety law?

5 Name the five classifications of fire extinguisher.

6 Name three factors that must be present to produce fire.

7 State three means of extinguishing a fire.

8 Which regulation relates to the need to report accidents in the
   workplace?

9 Name the three methods of sterilisation.

10 What does the acronym PPE stand for?

The answers to this activity can be found at the back of the book.

Assessment activity level B

Draw a plan of your salon. In the plan identify clearly:

- fire exits
- fire extinguishers.

Name the types of fire extinguishers in the salon.

Name the identified person/s in the salon responsible for:

- health and safety
- first aid.

Explain your salon's procedure for evacuating the salon in the case of an emergency.

Assessment activity level C

Produce a health and safety policy that includes:

- safe use of working methods and equipment
- safe use of hazardous substances
- smoking, eating, drinking and drugs
- what to do in the case of an emergency
- personal appearance and conduct.

The answers to these activity can be found at the end of the book.

Assessment activity level A: Word search

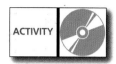

Word search

```
Q B X R G M A I N T E N A N C E Q G B K Q C K W E P G M B
M G L E V I T U C E X E Y T E F A S D N A H T L A E H A W
E P M E N W Y F P C E A W V T P M C I B P C J B A R P U H
S X J X B S U S X O B D I A T S R I F P G P P K T I Q M G
R G T Z P M O P O L I C Y H M R N Q O C O M X B Y K Q H V
R P S I L P T E Y D E B P U E S S H N B A F T M E A P A A
Y T Y N N B K Y Z H C X C G R I N X J H N X U N Q E O C B R
L P Q F D G P D M I Z J C T V J C G S E C N A T S B U S K
Q X C P R M U P T M Y X V Y R O H C U T V D R A Z A H H P
X T D O R V I I C R H E A L T H A N D S A F E T Y L A W N
L W Y R U J N I S W A Q S C E X E J H G N S K K C E G I T
H X Y L E U H J H H D I O N W P B B X Y C D K T V P K V M
D E R M A T I T I S E O N M E S K O C O N P G J E T N E Q
A D T B Q P I H M O T R A I K Z L C W S V Y A V E G K R G
N S J T C P Z U J M I V E J N N K G R Q E R J B Q R J Y V
B W Z O F U Y M U J H G T X L G C O U L H J S J V A U U O
L P E R S O N A L P R O T E C T I V E E Q U I P M E N T Q
F A B T A N N L P A S T E R I L E D R E S S I N G B X C V
V A C X P X G Y J M C S J E U N S M P Q X W P Z N P X Q P
R J P C T L N W I C A N H J Z N D G Y P J K Z E O V V M H
X Z E I I P F W K L G B E D R Y A R L Y O H Y G I L E T O
K W R O J D I X O C R T F Q I X L M L M I U Z X T M Q U X
B O I G E H E N G A L U Q J S F C H N A M U K Q A A P N S
Y O F U C N P N P V N J M U K B R F E U P N O E L M U U I
A H Y W E O V F T V B Y X F I Q B H L R D R U G S P D Z W
U Y H E L V U A Z B Z I T X I W K O N S E F D B I F E E X
K X A I E L P E R S O N A L H Y G I E N E M Z M G N F J A
S X C N G E T I K V P O R M E C P L G H I M T J E T K B H
C Y B R N O G E M W J C K S N O I T A L U G E R L D L F T
```

LEGISLATION	REGULATIONS
HEALTHANDSAFETYLAW	SUBSTANCES
PERSONALHYGIENE	DERMATITIS
PERSONALPROTECTIVEEQUIPMENT	SALONPOLICY
HAZARD	RISK
EXTINGUISHER	FIRSTAIDBOX
STERILEDRESSING	ACCIDENTBOOK
INJURY	FIRE
HEALTHANDSAFETYEXECUTIVE	TRAINING
POLICY	MAINTENANCE
DRUGS	

The answers to this activity can be found at the end of the book.

Assessment activity levels B and C: Crossword

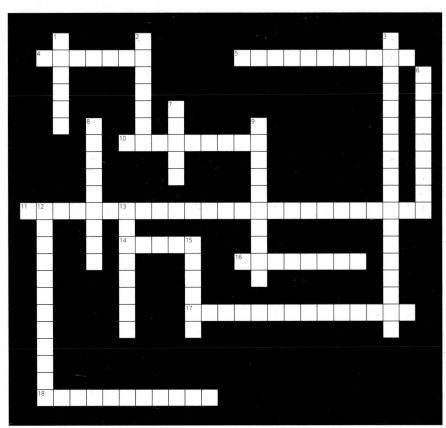

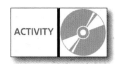

Crossword

Across
4. Personal behaviour
5. Collection of medical equipment (three words)
10. To let in fresh air
11. This organisation creates health and safety regulations (four words)
14. Abbreviation of the control of substances hazardous to health
16. Means to escape (two words)
17. Method of evaluating danger (two words)
18. Rules that govern procedure

Down
1. Health and safety criteria operated by the salon
2. Very clean
3. This needs to be a safe place (two words)
6. Blue liquid that sterilises tools
7. Do not use on electrical fires
8. When heat is transmitted without contact
9. Condition affecting the skin
12. Puts out fires
13. Mishap
15. This has a potential to cause harm

The answers to this activity can be found at the back of the book.

answers to assessment activities

Chapter 1

Assessment activity A

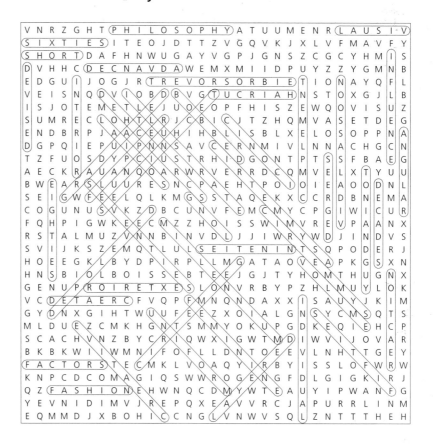

Assessment activity B

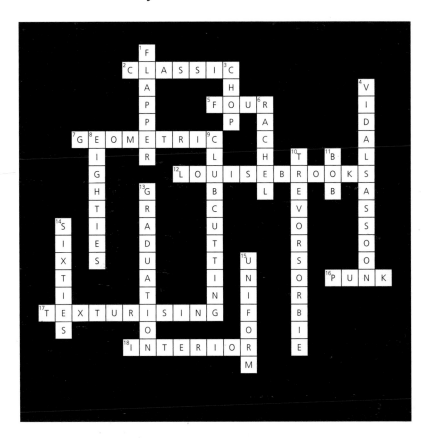

Chapter 2

Assessment activity level B

1 c eyelids
2 a vellus hair
3 b cuticle
4 a cortex
5 d vitamin D
6 d the hair to stand on end
7 c corneum
8 b sebum
9 a resting stage of the hair growth cycle
10 d type

Assessment activity level C

1 ● It is the outermost part of the hair.

 ● It is made up of overlapping layers of translucent scales.

 ● It has up to 11 layers of cuticle.

 ● The scales may be likened to tiles of a roof in the way that each lies over the other.

 ● The scales of the cuticle play an important part in the condition of the hair.

 ● Hair that is in good condition will have a cuticle that lies flat and is smooth.

 ● Uneven or broken cuticle layers lead to tangling of the hair and the lack of gloss makes the hair look dull.

2 ● Stratum corneum.

 ● Stratum lucidum.

 ● Stratum granulosum.

 ● Stratum spinosum.

 ● Stratum germinativum.

3 ● Protection.

 ● Absorption.

 ● Excretion and secretion.

 ● Temperature control.

 ● Sense of touch.

4 ● Anagen – Active hair growth lasting from 1.5 to 7 years. Nutrients provided by blood supply at dermal papilla.

 ● Catagen – Only lasts for around two weeks. New cell production ceases at the dermal papilla. The follicle begins to detach itself from the blood supply and begins to shrink away from the dermal papilla.

 ● Telogen – Complete resting stage of hair growth lasting for period of four months. At the end of the resting stage, the follicle re-attaches itself to the papilla and the blood supply once again supplies the nutrients to allow new hair growth, starting a new anagen stage.

5 ● Caucasian – Many different characteristics. It may be straight, wavy or curly, coarse or fine in texture, and may vary in colour from black to the palest blonde. Cross-section: oval.

 ● African type – Generally very curly, and often frizzy, but the type of curl can vary from soft and open to tight and woolly. Frequently brown, dark brown or black, but can also be red or blonde. Often very fine and delicate and easily damaged. Cross-section: flat.

 ● Asian – Includes the dark glossy hair that you associate with India or Pakistan, and the much straighter Oriental-type hair that can be found in the Far East – China and Japan. This type of hair grows much faster than that of Caucasian or African-type hair. Asian hair is often much coarser than Caucasian or African type. Cross-section: round.

Assessment activity level B

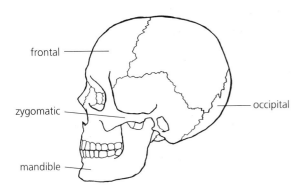

Assessment activity levels B and C

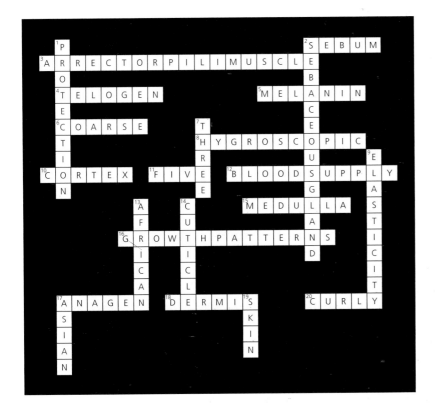

Assessment activity level A

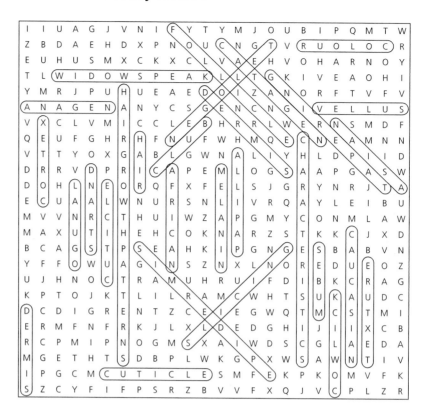

Chapter 3

Assessment activity level A

Condition	Infectious, contagious or non-infectious
Fragilitis crinium	non-infectious
Psoriasis	non-infectious
Sebaceous cyst	non-infectious
Alopecia areata	non-infectious
Head lice	contagious
Impetigo	infectious
Warts	infectious
Tinea capiti	infectious
Folliculitis	infectious
Trichorrhexis nodosa	non-infectious
Seborrhoea	non-infectious
Monilethrix	non-infectious
Scabies	infectious
Keloids	non-infectious
Damaged hair	non-infectious
Pityriasis capitis	non-infectious

Assessment activity level B

A Round
B Oval
C Long
D Heart/triangular
E Rectangular
F Pear
G Square
H Diamond

Assessment activity level B

1 The belief in the reliability of a person.

2 Being able to use all forms of communication effectively so that you are clearly understood.

3
- Speak clearly and unambiguously
- Vary voice tone and inflections
- Speak with courtesy and confidence
- Use professional vocabulary and not slang
- Never speak while you are eating or chewing gum

4
- Making an appointment or writing down a message
- Gestures and facial expressions
- Eye contact
- Clothes and accessories

5
- Body language
- Tone of voice
- Words

6
- Body language 50 per cent
- Tone of voice 40 per cent
- Words you use 10 per cent

7 A service in which the stylist asks the client questions to find out what the client wants and carries out an analysis of the client's hair and scalp.

8 Analysis is the term used for the checking of the hair and scalp for any disorders prior to a service. The purpose of analysis is to:
- decide on the most suitable cutting techniques to use to create the desired result
- decide on the most suitable cutting tools to use to achieve the desired result
- decide what products will be needed and advise the client
- advise the client on the maintenance requirements.

9 Avoid topics that are sensitive and could cause offence such as:
- religion
- racial remarks

- sex
- politics

10 Open questions can start with any one of the following words:

- who
- what
- where
- would
- when
- how.

Closed questions are used to gain a limited amount of response such as 'yes' and 'no'.

Assessment activity level B

Examples will vary according to your experiences.

Effective communication	Example of effective communication
Know the information and match your message to your audience	
Respect your client and reserve judgements	
Be mindful of what your body language is saying	
Listen carefully	
Stay focused and don't be distracted	
Be mindful of your tone of voice	
Think from your client's point of view	
Clarify information to ensure you and your client have understood each other	

Assessment activity levels B and C

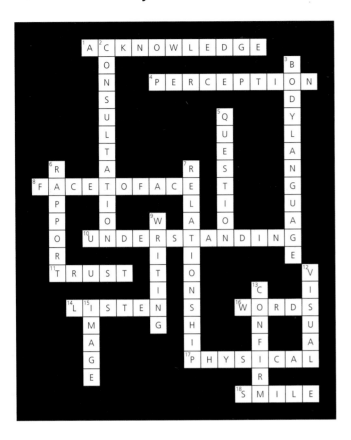

Chapter 4

Assessment of knowledge and understanding

1 Points of the blade, blades, blade edge, heel, pivot or screw system, shanks, handles

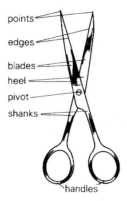

2 Only the thumb moves during the cutting process, allowing that blade to move against the second blade which remains still at all times.

3 Holds the blades in place and controls the tension on the scissors.

4 Handle, tang, heel, back and edge

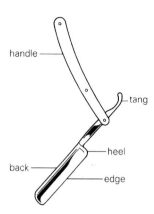

5 ● Heat = the use of an autoclave

   ● Radiation = the use of an ultraviolet light box

   ● Chemicals = the use of barbicide.

6 Heat – the autoclave.

7 Detachable clipper comb attachments enable the hair to be cut to a predetermined length.

8 Convex blades are the sharpest for slicing the hair.

9 To remove weight by tapering the ends of the hair or to create a textured effect.

10 When passing the razor make sure that the razor is closed, wrap your hand around the razor to prevent it from opening and pass the razor with the tang facing away from you but towards the person you are passing it to.

Assessment activity level B

1 Scissors.

2 Serrated.

3 Texturising.

4 Convex.

5 Pivot.

6 Tapering.

7 Sharps.

8 Radiation.

9 Environmental.

10 Recommend.

Assessment Activity Level A

1

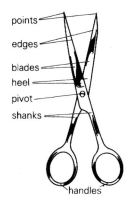

points
edges
blades
heel
pivot
shanks
handles

2

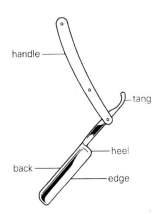

handle
tang
heel
back
edge

Assessment activity levels A and B

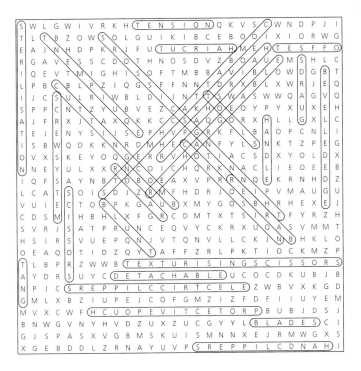

Assessment activity level C

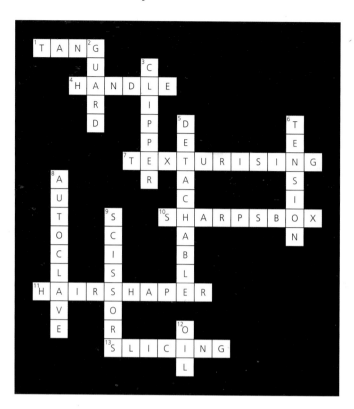

Chapter 5

Assessment activity level A

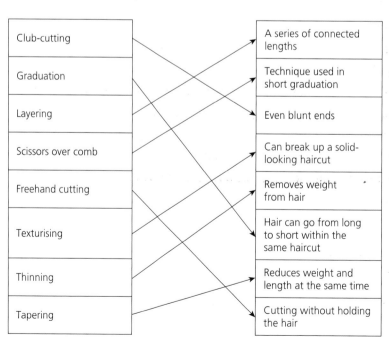

Club-cutting	A series of connected lengths
Graduation	Technique used in short graduation
Layering	Even blunt ends
Scissors over comb	Can break up a solid-looking haircut
Freehand cutting	Removes weight from hair
Texturising	Hair can go from long to short within the same haircut
Thinning	Reduces weight and length at the same time
Tapering	Cutting without holding the hair

Assessment activity level A

1 correct.

2 growth.

3 disconnected.

4 right angle.

5 hairline.

6 texturing.

7 freehand.

8 cowlick.

9 type.

10 forty-five degree.

Assessment activity level B

1 b hair cut to even lengths

2 c how curly the hair is

3 b non-serrated scissors

4 d freehand cutting

5 b hair too short

6 d guides

7 a disconnected

8 d lying flat

9 c long and angular

10 c temples

Assessment activity level C

1 Club-cutting.

2 The hair is not held with the hands, tools or equipment.

3 By curling the hair between the fingers before club-cutting.

4 Because you would create steps in a haircut or remove too much hair.

5 To create a guaranteed even length for the haircut.

6 A bob or one-length cut.

7 Length and weight removed at the same time.

8 Weight removed from the hair, but length remains the same.

9 A forerunner of fashion.

10 Any two from tapered, square, round.

Assessment activity levels A and B

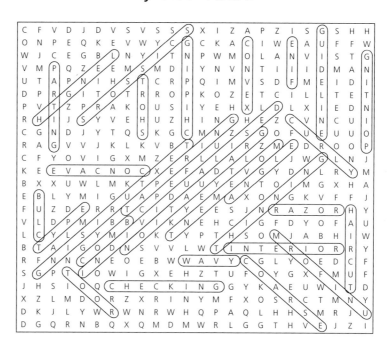

Assessment activity level C

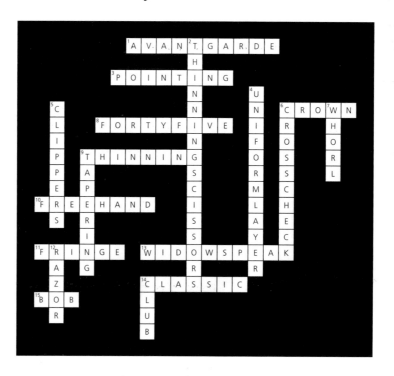

Chapter 7

1 Health and Safety at Work Act 1974.

2 A hazard is something with the potential to cause harm.

3 A risk is the likelihood of (someone being harmed by the hazard) the hazard's potential being realised.

4 Health and Safety Executive.

5
- Class A – solid, organic materials
- Class B – liquids
- Class C – gases
- Class D – metals
- Class F – liquefiable solids such as fats and cooking oils

6
- Fuel
- Oxygen
- Heat

7
- Cooling
- Starving
- Smothering

8 RIDDOR – Reporting of Injuries, Diseases and Dangerous Occurrences Regulations 1995.

9
- Heat
- Radiation
- Chemical

10 Personal protective equipment.

Assessment activity level A

Link the legislation on the left with the reason for the legislation on the right. Use may use different coloured markers to show your connections.

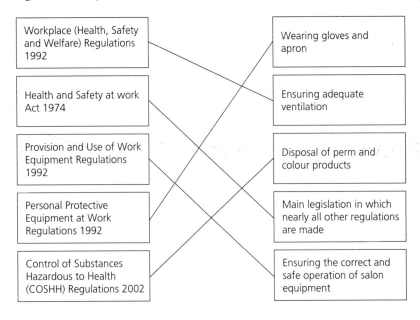

Assessment activity level A

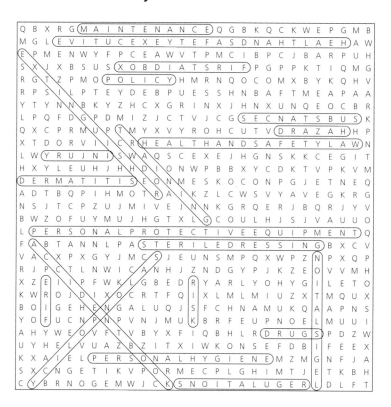

Assessment activity levels B and C

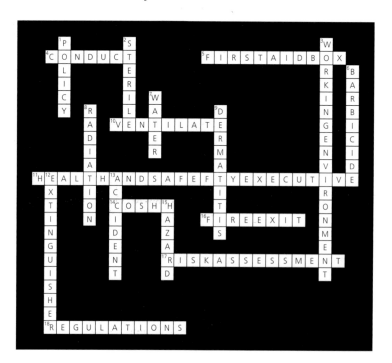

index

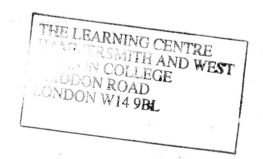